THE DUST BUSTING CHRONICLES

CHRONICLES

Cleaning My Way Through Ovarian Cancer

Cheryl L. Cushine

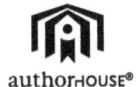

authorHOUSE®

AuthorHouse™
1663 Liberty Drive, Suite 200
Bloomington, IN 47403
www.authorhouse.com
Phone: 1-800-839-8640

First published by AuthorHouse 6/29/2007

ISBN: 978-1-4343-1285-3 (e)
ISBN: 978-1-4343-1284-6 (sc)
ISBN: 978-1-4343-2167-1 (hc)

Printed in the United States of America
Bloomington, Indiana

This book is printed on acid-free paper.

DEDICATED TO THOSE WHOSE GRACE AND
KINDNESS IS THEIR OFFERING, THE SWEET ROSE
PERFUME OF THEIR BEING.

CHERYL L. CUSHINE

CONTENTS

Chapter One: One Ending, One Beginning   1

Chapter Two: It's Probably Nothing Serious   6

Chapter Three: All About the Tests   14

Chapter Four: It Really is Cancer   31

Chapter Five: Finding Our Way   42

Chapter Six: Down to a Science   67

Chapter Seven: Keep On Keepin' On   99

Chapter Eight: It Is What It Is   121

CHAPTER ONE:
ONE ENDING, ONE BEGINNING

I was leaving the ghosts and goblins behind. As I checked my rearview mirror for anything left in the driveway, I could see them, all of them—the ghouls of chemotherapy and the goblins of hair loss and nausea—dangling from the porch we used to jam with brilliant seasonal flowers and holiday ceramics—the porch where we relished steaming mugs of coffee and thick Sunday papers.

To shake the phantoms, I had to abandon the home we had shared for eight idyllic years—the home with the cozy oak trimmed kitchen wafting molasses-laced pot roast and carrots; the home with warm antiques and gentle lighting; the home of generous meals, full-bodied wines and gracious hospitality; the home that felt like a sanctuary to all who entered.

She had passed from cancer six months earlier, on April 25, 2004. I knew, shortly after her death, that my life in New Jersey was over. The safe and cozy world I had known had been snuffed out like a tea light, choked by its own wax. My world looked uninviting, dingy, and foreign. I had to rebuild my life in a place that wasn't being rented to the ghosts and goblins floating behind me.

1

During our two-year battle with ovarian cancer, the living room couch transformed from snug loveseat to chemo-recovery divan sporting a vomit bin, crusty tissues, and saltine cracker crumbs. Overnight, our cozy bed draped with a handmade quilt and crisp pink cotton sheets became a place for painful dry-heaving, nightmares, and infusion-induced comas that were the sleep of death.

From the bed, Lyse watched as I dressed for work in the mornings. She was in no hurry to get up. Death was coming whether she was up or not. She'd smile at me lazily as I watched the sunlight from the arc window brush across her pale face and cracked lips. Then it danced in her fading brown eyes, and settled onto her shiny scalp that had retained a couple of thin, wispy hairs.

The master bath, once our passion spa, had changed from a place of steamy showers and lovemaking to an agonizing repository of retch, diarrhea, and eventually, small, hard feces forced through intestines blocked by a black, cancerous growth.

No, I couldn't stay in River Edge. I couldn't even stay in New Jersey. I quit my corporate job, sold our beloved home, and packed the car for Wilmington, North Carolina. I sort of figured that the ghosts and goblins wouldn't bother chasing me 600 miles to the south. I wasn't too sure, though.

On Halloween day, 2004, I drove into Wilmington. It was warm and sunny, and there wasn't a ghost in sight. It felt safe and nurturing. I had driven from the tomb to the womb. I was feeling better already. Maybe, I could pull it together—build a new life for myself, and see fewer of those phantoms hanging on the Jordan Drive porch.

"I'm not crappin' ya, Cher. It's freaking awesome down here in Dixieland," my friend, Sue, had gushed over the phone a month after the funeral.

"You know," she lingered, misshapen Boston vowels quashing her sentences, "Eileen and I are pigs in shit down here—mild weather, the ocean and the Cape Fear River around the corner, low, low taxes...and southern cooking—you know, hush puppies, grits, and gravy smothered over everything! You gotta come down."

She had sampled and rated the hush puppies all over town, from Elijah's Seafood to the Sawmill Restaurant down in Monkey Junction, modeled after kitchens in North Carolina logging camps circa 1930. The small oval blobs of fried, sweet cornbread yielded a flavorful, chewy dough with bits of satisfying sticky corn.

My belly button was buzzing. Grief or no grief, my gut had trumpeted the time for a complete life turnaround. Wilmington proper, a city of almost 100,000, covets an impressive Civil War history, southern charm in its antebellum mansions, solid art museums and theatre, downtown shopping, waterfront beauty, and an influx of northerners seeking a more tranquil existence.

"Mother Mary told me Wilmington was the place," Sue explained excitedly. "I asked her where Eileen and I needed to be next, and she placed my hand over Wilmington on the map. I'm tellin' ya, there's a vortex here—an incredible energy. Pennsylvania's for the birds."

Her connection to Mother Mary and other spiritual beings like the Dalai Lama ran deep. I would come to connect more pragmatically with the soothing timbres of the river and ocean, no thanks to a mystical map or swirling eddy.

No one agreed with my plan.

"The general wisdom is that one should wait at least a year before making any decisions," my stepdad, Sidney, counseled. The psychiatrist in him peered at me through the telephone line, disapprovingly, over the top of his tortoise shell rims.

The general wisdom has typically run a close second to the acumen of my navel.

Each night after work I packed. I put yellow stickers on boxes with Lyse's stuff, green stickers on my stuff to be stored, and orange stickers on boxes of things that were Wilmington-bound. Molly, my four-and-a-half pound Yorkie, was puzzled and agitated by the packing tape, musty boxes, and my zeal. Leftover caregiver adrenaline, discomfort from the basement's glaring light bulbs and a cold, cement floor spurred me on night-after-night for three months until the job was done.

The belongings I would need for my four-month stay at the Main Stay Suites—a pet-friendly, budget hotel on Wilmington's congested downtown strip, included: laptop, clothing, Molly's toys and couch, a small pouch of good jewelry, Bose CD/radio, important papers like the contract for my pre-construction town home, Grandma's Limoges vase, and Lyse's silver letter opener—a gift from her parochial school kids in 1971. A southwestern bowl stuffed with potpourri, two bright throw rugs, and my own blue and white striped bedding completed the mix, and warmed the first floor room.

Moving to Wilmington was the easy part. Getting the ghouls out of my mind would take some doing. Thoughts of ditching it—my corporate job, our Dickensian neighborhood, and solid friends—had plagued me from the moment I left the funeral home. My new path was clearly marked and I intuitively knew to climb aboard. Without Lyse, I was anchorless—heaviness and buoyancy, intertwined in paradox, one because of the other. The paradox was creating energy for change, and it had me by the throat. I was ready.

Three Halloweens later, I was living a peaceful and contented life in Wilmington, mostly free of ghouls. Molly had since passed. All ties to my old life had vanished. My soul connection to Lyse and Molly, however, transcending physical boundaries, was impervious to time and earthly limitations. I was filled with complete peace in that realization. Love was eternal, and would not be bound by the frailties of our bodies, our homes, our wedding rings, or other incidental memorabilia.

Lyse and I had been visited by two rabbits the night we shared our first kiss, at a panoramic esplanade above the Hudson River in Englewood, New Jersey. Nine years later, the evening I scattered her ashes on the shores of North Carolina's Outer Banks, our beloved vacation spot, I was visited by one rabbit. He turned to look at me, and watched as the wind carried the soft remains, and deposited them into a bed of salt marsh. He hopped away, gracefully, toward the tall reeds, and then turned slowly to gaze at me, with gentle brown eyes, one last time.

The sky turned to night.

CHAPTER TWO:
IT'S PROBABLY NOTHING SERIOUS

Wednesday, September 11, 2002

"I'm going to need surgery," Lyse said, matter-of-factly from her seat on the couch.

She sat on the right end cushion—the one Molly stretched out on at night while we watched television. She wore a blue crewneck sweater and jeans from Lands End. She was a size 14 and had pointed out to me several times that she used to be a size 12, but in her fifties, "things had headed south." She had accepted this migration, mostly the changes around her middle, and told me, "each decade has its own beauty," in spite of the body's unfortunate changes.

She loved crewneck sweaters and had one in every color of the rainbow. They made her look collegiate and professorial, like a New Englander. She was.

"They found fluid on my ovaries and I know that's not good. They're going to have to get the fluid out," she continued, in what I recognized as her authoritative teacher's voice—the one she used to get the kids' attention in class.

Her eyes were intent and focused on me. I could sense her fear, which was turbulent beneath her stoic words, like a wave of nausea before throwing up.

I had just returned home from work. Once home, I routinely kissed Lyse, and then lifted Mol's wriggling frame high into the air and to my face. She would cover me in kisses with an elongated tongue, which we swore belonged to an anteater. That day, I kissed Molly and then walked over to the couch where Lyse sat, her back rigid and feet flat on the floor.

The one thing I couldn't do fast enough, once I got home, was get out of my work clothes. After ten hours in an airtight, stuffy office building, my foundation and blush had usually retreated to reveal a splotchy, sallow complexion. My dried-up contact lenses barely clung to my reddened eyes, and my French braid had mutated from a shiny style to a shellacked clump. I called it "getting changed." Lyse called it "changing up."

A French Canadian by birth, with time spent living in Providence, Rhode Island and the Bronx, New York, Lyse had culled an interesting mix of accents and colloquialisms. Lyse's sister, who was eleven years older, had managed to hang onto her accent completely. It was pleasant to hear Jeannine say just about anything, as she stretched vowels and elongated consonants, lilting all the way.

"No matter what it is, babe, we're going to get through it," I remember saying, somewhat sternly, as if my forcefulness could will away the dark clouds coming our way.

"You're right, I know," she responded quietly. Her voice was raspy.

I took her left hand and mindlessly twirled her commitment ring, the same as mine, a handmade circle of braided gold. We had them custom made in New Hope, Pennsylvania, five months after our first date at Barnes & Noble, May 3, 1996. Soul mates we were. Life partners we became.

"Dr. Huss said my blood work showed high liver counts. He also said the CA 125 count is abnormal and the pelvic sonogram showed fluid on the ovaries," she continued.

For the past twenty years, Lyse had faithfully seen the silver-haired, old-school Dr. Huss annually, for a gynecologic exam that included blood work with a CA 125 test—a cancer antigen marker test that indicates the presence of ovarian cancer—and a routine pap smear. Due to a history of ovarian cancer in the family—Lyse's sister, Georgette, had passed from the disease at age sixty—Dr. Huss also required that Lyse have her ovaries checked for any change in size. There had been no change to the ovaries that year. However, because of Lyse's elevated liver counts and an elevated CA 125 marker, Dr. Huss scheduled her for a pelvic sonogram right away.

Results of the sonogram, held September 10, 2002, as reported by Dr. Noah Weg, indicated "mildly increased fluid in the cul-de-sac" and no visualization of the right ovary.

"Let's wait until we have all the necessary information before jumping to conclusions, sweetie," I offered soothingly.

I didn't change up until bedtime that day.

Friday, September 13, 2002

A transvaginal pelvic sonogram, the next diagnostic step, will be performed today. Dr. Weg's follow-up report indicated "echogenic fluid in the right adnexa suggesting some complex fluid in the region."

Summer of that year had been good. Our time together always was. We had vacationed on Block Island, Rhode Island, in July, and had spent an overnight in historic Lambertville, New Jersey during my birthday weekend in August. Looking back at pictures from those trips, I see bloating, and a bit of pallidness throughout Lyse's angelic face. Her eyes—my eyes are always the first to betray me when fatigue or stress is running high—were smaller than usual, dull, and devoid of their usual sparkle. I examined those pictures, and others of us back then, and felt sorry for the people, knowing what laid ahead for them.

Life is hard whether one is in love or just loving. With Lyse, I came to understand the not so subtle difference between the two. I also came to a realization that the other partners in my life had been people I merely loved. It's not that loving isn't good enough. It's rather perfect between certain people. The difference, I discovered, was all about the giving—the kind of giving that never ends and doesn't keep track.

Giving of oneself spiritually, sexually, mentally and emotionally—all four, no less. It means caring more about bestowing those gifts than what or how much is given. It's also about the connection one feels. It's less like a salt and pepper duo and more like the mortar-pestle thing.

Lyse was a regular customer at the Barnes & Noble café on Friday nights. She'd leisurely sip her café latte while browsing computer and science magazines. She would sneak peeks at me while I was playing flute next to my guitarist, up front near the Linzer tarts and napoleons.

Lyse and I had come to know each other through mutual friends. We'd happen upon each other at teacher get-togethers, like dinners out and Super Bowl parties. Our conversations were limited and few, but were interspersed with many intoxicating smiles. She gazed from a distance, quietly and discreetly.

She began admiring the café flutist after her partner left. A proud but humble, loyal and steadfast woman, Lyse suffered a major blow from the breakup. A friendship that had spanned twenty-five years and had been birthed in the convent had ended abruptly. Lyse was stunned and wounded deeply, but through it all, she had maintained a solid sense of self-preservation and an ability to heal herself.

During that time, she often thought about what her mother, a victim of kidney cancer, had told her years earlier about the ups and downs of life. She helped explain her husband's squalls and what they were doing to the family: "Everyone in life gets their black bread and their white bread. You're getting your black bread first. Down the road, it will be better."

Lyse had entered the convent when she was a dewy, eighteen year old. She wanted to help the world as a nurse or a teacher. After trying on her sister's nurse's cap and being scolded for tempting bad luck, she opted for the career with more favorable odds.

Eighteen years in the convent had allowed Lyse to fulfill her dream of spiritual-based world change—for a while, anyway. By the time she spoke with Mother Superior, Lyse knew that she'd have to continue her calling to teach, but in civilian clothes. Life in the convent had been a joy. Lyse prayed, chanted and studied scripture. She changed lives in school systems from the Bronx to Rhode Island. She sipped a beer or two and sang to Motown with the other girls at the Friday night dances. A cigarette up on the roof wasn't out of the question, either. I was always surprised and relieved to know that the girls of prayer knew how to have fun, perhaps even better than the rest of us.

Lyse had an incredible depth of spirit, as well as a mischievous one. She won people over with her kindness and gentleness. The statue of Mother Mary even acquiesced as Lyse hid the box of shared cigarettes under her concrete skirt.

Lyse eventually moved through civilian life resourcefully, accomplishing in eighteen years what most people did in twice that time. She owned a home, and had become a science department chair in Tenafly—an upscale and progressive New Jersey school district. She was well liked and exceedingly talented.

By the time I knocked on the door of Lyse's life, she had resigned herself to the fact that a spinster existence would claim her in the end. I saved her from that fate, but in the process, wove an interesting destiny for myself.

We all have primal hopes and primal needs. We mostly hide them and usually take them to the grave unfulfilled. It's sort of like having a couple of old Post-it-notes still hanging on the fridge at the time of one's passing.

Some of us are astute enough to realize the point in time when we're awarded the chance to fulfill our primal longings. They consist of desires, hopes, and needs that are buried so far down that we've lost touch with them—desires and needs so great that they make or break our happiness. How many of us can recognize them, tap into them, and hoist them up far enough to actually greet them even *when* we feel safe with another human being and are loved unconditionally?

I could, with Lyse. I wanted to, with Lyse. I did, with Lyse. She made it comfortable for me to meet myself on the other side, and feel things that only a soul mate could help one do.

And she did it intuitively.

Wednesday, September 18, 2002

Lyse was scheduled for an abdominal sonogram today. Dr. Weg's report would later conclude that, "ascites is noted, unknown etiology. The examination is otherwise unremarkable."

I learned that ascites means "fluid" and wondered why they just didn't call it that on the report. Ascites is the presence of fluid in the peritoneal cavity—

11

the abdominal cavity containing organs such as the stomach, liver, bowels, spleen, uterus, ovaries, and fallopian tubes—and is lined by a membrane called the peritoneum.

Sidney called that night to talk to Lyse. For a few minutes, she mostly listened and murmured, and would occasionally say, "Thank you," and "I really appreciate your concern."

Mom and Sidney adored Lyse. Her gentle demeanor, unadulterated concern for others, and the way she took care of me endeared her to them. They enjoyed her company. She and Mom shared recipes. She and Sidney swapped birding stories.

"Sidney said it's probably nothing serious," she said after hanging up. "He said, who knows, maybe a cyst has burst, or something like that, and not to jump to conclusions before all the data is in," she went on, her voice slightly brighter.

"I think that's good advice," I replied lightly. "Let's just take this one step at a time."

Regarding health, finances and safety, Sidney was typically an alarmist, always assuming the worst in every situation. He erred on the side of caution, and was a master planner for every catastrophe looming on the horizon. I was surprised at the hopefulness and optimism he displayed that night, considering his astuteness as a physician, and proclivity for pessimism.

The new school year was well underway and Lyse thought the kids were a good bunch. Many of the kids in the upper-crust Tenafly, New Jersey school district were high-achievers. Its education system was known far and wide for its excellence. Families from Japan and Korea spread the word back home. The next year, new kids came to Tenafly while their fathers conducted business in the states for a year or two.

"I really don't like missing school, especially at the beginning of the year like this," Lyse said slowly, with aching discomfort bathing her voice.

"I know, babe, but your health comes first," I responded gently. "Without that, you're no good to anyone."

She sighed and I hugged her tightly. I pressed into her and ran my fingers through her wavy, silver hair, enjoying its thickness and sweet smell.

CHAPTER THREE:
ALL ABOUT THE TESTS

Thursday, September 19, 2002

The Mayo Clinic, on its web site, mayoclinic.com, defines a CT scan—or CAT scan—as an "X-ray [*sic*] technique that produces images of your internal organs that are more detailed than those produced by conventional X-ray [*sic*] exams."

This technology allows the doctor to see cross-sections of the body, as opposed to the more conventional x-ray that only provides a two-dimensional image.

Lyse complained mildly about the infusion of dye she received since it felt warm and "funny" inside her, moving around on its own. She mistakenly thought she had urinated on the table when she felt the penetrating, sudden warmth in her groin. Plus, the table was cold and uncomfortable. Other than that, she said it wasn't too bad.

Dr. Weg's radiology report to Dr. Huss described, "a moderate amount of ascites present throughout the abdomen and pelvis. There is infiltration of the omentum. Although not specific, this finding is most frequently associated with malignant ascites."

The omentum is a fatty fold of the peritoneum that surrounds the stomach and other abdominal organs.

❦

Lyse cooked every night. She was usually home from school around 4:00 p.m., except on the days when she had faculty or departmental meetings. She enjoyed searching for new recipes in magazines or on the Internet. Jeannine routinely sent her innovative and healthy meal ideas.

The recipe box I gave her for Christmas 1998 is painted like a birdhouse. There is a pink roof, and the front and sides of the house are speckled with bright flowers in pink, blue, purple and yellow. Together, we created the categories we needed: pasta, beef, chicken, pork, potatoes, soup, vegetables, casseroles, appetizers, bread, and desserts. The birdhouse today remains stuffed with our findings, such as, Garden Vegetable Soup, Swiss Turkey Quiche—written on the back of a hall pass—Red Bean and Rice Soup, and Hurry-Up Meat Loaves.

Arriving home from work on any given day, I might inhale savory aromas such as Mediterranean Chicken simmered in tomatoes and topped with pimento olives, green peppers stuffed with low-fat beef, cubed tomatoes, chili spice and cheddar cheese, flavorful white bean and rosemary soup, or steaming pasta smothered with creamy garlic-herb cheese and tomato slices.

The kitchen was an intimate nook. A tiny oak table—a bargain from IKEA—sat in front of the window that looked out on our neighborhood—a demographically diverse community of forty-five homes. Lyse enjoyed the view and would often sit, tea mug in hand, watching neighbors unload groceries, plant flowers, or play ball with their kids.

The townhouse spanned 1,900 square feet. Built in 1988, the home boasted three bathrooms, hardwood floors, open living room and dining room, wood-burning fireplace, two bedrooms, garage and basement. Cathedral ceilings in both bedrooms lent a dramatic flair to the rooms. An arc window in the master bedroom created an enchanting niche on the far wall. We relished our furnishings of oriental rugs over wood floors, dark French-Colonial style furniture and fabrics of steel blue, mauve, sage and plum. We delighted in the warmth and safety of our little sanctuary. We had quickly assumed domestic life together and adjusted with ease.

Friday, September 20, 2002

Things were moving quickly. Based upon the results of Lyse's CT scan, Dr. Huss immediately referred her to Dr. Gennauoi, who was working out of Good Samaritan Hospital in Suffern, New York. A non-profit hospital with approximately 370 beds, the hospital offers a range of services including emergency, medical, surgical and obstetrical. It serves residents of northern Bergen County, New Jersey as well as Rockland and southern Orange counties in New York. I took off a personal half-day from work. We drove up Route 17 into Rockland County, then down Route 59, toward the hospital for our 2:00 p.m. meeting with the surgeon.

Friday afternoons were electrifying—everyone beholding the weekend in jovial giddiness with time to play, sleep in, or eat out. All of the cars on the road that afternoon streaked toward their weekend destinations. I could sense the intoxication of the drivers as they anticipated their impending downtime—the change of pace for two short days. I was excited, too. Adrenaline about our upcoming battle had filled every corner of my being, and had me pumped up like a heavyweight before entering the ring. I was fortified and ready. I was going into combat against this foe with Lyse, beside her, and for her. I would lift her up.

"Did you eat lunch, baby?" I asked hopefully, steering through the winding roads between Route 17 and Route 59.

I had gulped a homemade peanut butter on wheat sandwich during my six mile commute home from work.

"No, I wasn't hungry and can't even think about eating right now," she replied absent-mindedly, staring out the window at the reds and oranges of the trees, just beginning their yearly transition.

"You've got to keep something in your stomach, sweetie, a little bit so you don't get light-headed," I answered softly.

I veered into Eckerd Drugs on Route 59. The setup to get to the parking lot was screwy. I maneuvered Lyse's navy Saab hatchback through a skinny driveway, around the building, and then into the front where we entered a parking lot filled with tight, uneven spaces. I felt nettled and antagonized by the ridiculous layout of the place. Parking quickly and jumping out of the car, I could feel the knot in my neck, the tension in my upper spine. I walked briskly. My dress boots clomped the pavement, and my gabardine cuffed slacks slid up and down my legs. I searched the cracker and cookie aisle for something light and easy for Lyse to eat. I picked up a jumbo-sized bag of Combos, pretzels stuffed with cheese.

Hmmmm. She really likes these. She can't lose weight before the battle has even started. She can't go into surgery skin and bones.

I paid for the pretzels and hurried back to the car. I opened the bag to tempt her, and she reluctantly picked out two. We headed toward the hospital.

"You're going to need surgery right away, to remove the fluid and determine exactly what is going on," Dr. Gennauoi explained. "We will debulk what we can and take biopsies at that time," he continued.

My eyes were drawn to his bald, gleaming head and kind face. He was a short man, perhaps in his early sixties, and exuded a comforting blend of professionalism and concern.

He had just completed a brief exam and re-read the results of Lyse's recent tests. He and Dr. Huss would jointly perform the abdominal and gynecologic surgery. A hysterectomy and removal of the infected peritoneum was planned.

"You'll be admitted to the hospital on Monday, and we'll do surgery on Wednesday, the twenty-fifth," he continued matter-of-factly and temperately.

Mom's birthday is Wednesday. That'll be good luck for Lyse.

Lyse nodded in agreement as Dr. Gennauoi spoke. She sat, unmoving, on the exam table, listened intently, and didn't take her eyes off the doctor. He explained that she would have an endoscopy—a procedure to examine the esophagus, stomach and upper part of the small intestine—and a colonoscopy on the Tuesday before surgery, as a way to address other possible conditions.

"We'll see you Monday, then. We'll take good care of you. Don't worry," Dr. Gennauoi said reassuringly as we headed out the door toward the car.

That night we baked a Tree Tavern frozen pizza, as we always did on Fridays.

"Thank you, Lord, for this day, and the many blessings in our lives. We ask for guidance and strength as we move forward at this time of uncertainty. Please give us courage as we go into surgery and deal with the outcome that is presented. Help us remember to return the blessings in our lives by remembering those around us. Thank you for our home, our relationship and our little Miss Molly," Lyse slowly recited our dinnertime prayer. Her voice quivered but there were no tears.

Although Lyse and I didn't attend church, we were both deeply spiritual. We believed it was more important to live our spirituality in each moment of each day, rather than committing to Sunday services because it was what everyone else did.

Lyse picked at her slice of pizza. I ate fervently. The crunch of the crust temporarily eased the whirl of thoughts and anxieties that assaulted my mind. My agitated metabolism had burned off the peanut butter sandwich hours ago. I picked up my glass of Merlot and slowly inhaled its fruity bouquet. I took a long sip, and let the velvety liquid swirl around my tongue and cheeks. I swallowed, enjoying the sensation, and then felt a knot of tension throb way back in my throat.

We spoke softly about the impending surgery and decided we wouldn't cross bridges we hadn't yet reached.

Monday, September 23, 2002

It was time to leave for the hospital. I had gone to work that morning and assigned my open tasks to my project management staff. Even though my team was completely competent, I worried about being out of the loop and slicing into what little paid time off I had stockpiled. I wanted to keep work and home smooth and flawless, and maintain a seamlessness in all areas of my life, especially now. Fairly new to my management role at work, I had felt it crucial to keep the impact from personal issues to a minimum.

Lyse picked at her egg sandwich, tossed it in the garbage, and then gathered her bags for the six-day hospital stay. That morning, I stuffed a love-note into Lyse's sweatshirt and another into the book she was reading by the Dalai Lama—*An Open Heart, Practicing Compassion in Everyday Life.* I had set up a revolving-door care team. Jeannine would be with us September 30 through October 5, which was perfect for week one. She'd spent a career in nursing—obstetrics and operating room recovery—and could provide the type of intimate care Lyse would require immediately after the hysterectomy and abdominal surgery. Monique, Lyse's youngest sister, would stay from October 13 through 18, and my mom would be here in-between both of them.

Unbeknown to me at the time, I would come to need Mom for emotional support by October 5. She would come to glimpse the beginnings of my self-destruction, as only a mother could.

Lyse and I worked our way through a lengthy admissions process, answered a copious amount of questions and provided no fewer than five clerks with documents such as Lyse's insurance card, supplemental insurance card, and driver's license. Each clerk sat at a desk with a cubicle, opposite the patients. We worked our way down the line of cubicles, and exchanged polite greetings with each teller. Unaware of the nightmare that awaited us, they were cheery, and bantered coolly with each other. Someone giggled. Everyone was very efficient as duplicate and triplicate copies of forms were printed. I was distracted and encouraged by the commotion and goodwill, which made me wonder if we had much to worry about after all.

Yellow, blue and white papers began to accumulate in my hand. At the last desk, we offered copies of Lyse's living will and power of attorney. The clerk looked surprised but not shocked. Many people mistook us for mother and daughter.

In 1999, Lyse and I began discussing our wishes with each other and felt it would be wise to formalize our intentions. On October 19, 2001, Lyse and I initialed our last will and testament documents with Deb Guston, a partner in Guston and Guston, LLP, Glen Rock, New Jersey. We both desired that no extreme medical measures be taken in the event of a terminal illness or life-threatening situation—no breathing machines, and nothing that would prolong an otherwise dire prognosis. Our estates were willed to each other, with the understanding that family heirlooms such as jewelry, dishes, and pictures, would be given to the appropriate relative.

We felt very comfortable and relieved that we had documented everything, and had defined every wish in clear terms. Doing so provided a safe harbor. It was a way of protecting each other and insured that our wishes were abided by, forever.

To celebrate our accomplishment that day, we went out to lunch at a small Italian place in Fair Lawn, New Jersey, and enjoyed Merlot with hearty bowls of pasta.

A smiling hospital volunteer took us to Lyse's room later that morning. I unpacked her duffel bag and methodically laid her book, nail file, eyeglass case, notebook and crossword puzzles on the bed tray. I placed her Land's End sweatpants, extra sweatshirt, two pair of underwear and three pair of Depends—"special underwear" as Lyse referred to them—in the bureau. I opened the closet door, hung her bag on the large hook and deposited her loafers on the floor.

I walked around Lyse's bed. To my surprise, my clogs made noise, just like crinkled cellophane, each time I lifted my foot.

The floor of the room is sticky. I can't believe this. Sh**. This is gross. Don't they mop the floors? Is this someone else's urine sticking to my shoes? Ugh!

I was completely hyped, angered, and consumed by the stickiness. My breathing caught and ratcheted up and down—clickety clack—in spasm.

How can the surgery be any good if the floors are sticky? Is there time to move her to a better hospital?

I was overwhelmed by everything that was turning sour, and seemed to be going wrong.

The floor nurse came to check Lyse's vital signs. She greeted Lyse pleasantly, and then called the janitor, who was wheeling his squeaky, yellow, dirt-streaked bucket down the hall. She instructed him to clean the dirty floor. She was annoyed also. His unsightly bucket tarnished the reputation of the entire hospital at that moment.

After the floor was mopped, I sat next to Lyse's bed and held her hand. There was little to say. We sat quietly for a moment.

I gazed at the single pink rose in a delicate vase that sat on the windowsill. The sprightly, coiffed-hair saleslady in the gift shop that afternoon was cheerful and very eager to help me pick out the perfect posy. Oddly, I found her merriness comforting—the antithesis of the heaviness I carried within. Lyse glanced at the vase also and thanked me again for such a beautiful flower. She smiled at me and her eyes, for a moment, brightened.

That evening, Lyse's nephew, Bob, visited from Westchester, New York. His wife, Sandra, had baked a large pan of lasagna for us.

Where will I put this in the freezer? So much stuff in there already. Ugh.

Gentle, mischievous and kindhearted, Bob had maintained a close relationship with his "Tante Lyse"—the French Canadian address—throughout his thirty-plus years. I greeted him at the door around 6:30 p.m. and was suddenly conscious of fatigue that gave my face a stretched-out feeling and caused my eyes to sway in sockets that had suddenly expanded.

In preparation for the bowel cleansing for the next day's procedures, the nurse had stationed a gray and white commode-on-wheels next to Lyse's bed. The action arrived when Bob showed up. The two managed to eke out a few pleasantries in-between calls of nature and acrobatics in and out of the bed, but the visit was cut short. Lyse felt badly about the outcome but just smiled.

With a weary shrug, she said, "It is what it is."

I walked with Bob out to the parking lot. I hugged him, put the frozen lasagna in the trunk of the car, and drove to Walgreen's to buy some more special underwear. It would be a long night for Lyse after I left for home.

My heart raced as I breezed down Route 17 south toward home, through Ramsey, past the Kawasaki dealer and Prestige BMW. Further along, I entered Paramus and passed the Burlington Coat store and Service Merchandise, along with numerous fast-food restaurants and signs for Paramus Park Mall. I was energized from overtiredness. I hummed to Stevie Nick's, *Leather and Lace.* The volume was way up. After a few bars, my stomach suddenly lurched and dropped. A beautiful turn in the melody snagged my brief respite. The tender tune reached down into my gut. It gently tickled and tantalized my sadness. It teased my anguish until it spurt. Then it gushed like a geyser swooshing the back of my throat and eyes until the hot tears came down my cheeks. They tasted salty on my lips. I continued driving, and was now solemn and heavy-hearted.

Monique and Jeannine will be here the day after tomorrow. Jeannine will be edgy and overwrought. I feel so responsible for everything. It's terrifying. I've got to keep going. So much to do now. A glass of brandy, kisses from Molly and my sleeping pills will be so good once I get home.

Finally, pulling into the garage, I sat quietly for a moment. My ears were ringing and my pulse pounded in my temples. I remembered the lasagna in the trunk.

One more thing I have to do. Goddamned noodles.

Tuesday, September 24, 2002

The endoscopy and colonoscopy would be done today. I was scheduled to meet with Dr. Alfred Hollander, after Lyse's procedure, to discuss the results. During my drive up to the hospital, I pondered the weather.

It always seemed that times of trouble or illness in one's life coincided with truly spectacular weather. Days when I've been home sick from work with a migraine or bad cold have typically been some of the nicest days of the year. It had always seemed like a cruel joke. During those times, when I was angry about this, Lyse helped me to focus on what *was* rather than what I thought things should be. She pointed out, reassuringly, that things are the way they should be at a particular point in time. Her philosophy of, "it is what it is" transformed my ability to accept things as they are, and to not waste energy or create negativity by being angry about life events as they naturally occur.

Before leaving the house this morning, I had straightened up more rigorously than usual. After doing the breakfast dishes, vacuuming the kitchen floor, foyer and flight of Italian-tile stairs leading from the basement to the foyer—the tile drew dust and dirt like a magnet—I went upstairs to the second floor and eyed Lyse's desk that sat on the far wall of our bedroom. Her Yorkie desk calendar was open to the week of September 22 with "Admitted to Hospital" splashed across Monday, the twenty-third. Her silver letter opener—engraved with, "Sr. Lyse, With gratitude from St. Joan's parishioners, June 1971"—laid in-between the calendar and a stack of medical and school papers that had started to tilt left from its own weight and bulk.

The crooked papers bothered me. I was conscious of the clock and my impending commute to the hospital. Northern Bergen County rush hour was truly the worst. Accidents were just waiting to happen in many cases. All of the main roads in our area—Routes 3, 4, 80/95, 17, and 46—were jammed each weekday with commuters fighting their way into Manhattan via the George Washington Bridge and Lincoln Tunnel, or traveling to various corporate complexes toward Totowa and west.

My breathing hastened. I gathered all the papers and tapped the cumbersome pile down on the desk. Then I separated it into smaller piles to tap so all the papers would be even. Symmetry was critical. Symmetry in my physical environment spawned peace in my being. Rest came only after I had cleaned and organized. Order, symmetry and cleanliness have always helped me cope with the blows and hardships of life. A neat home enabled me to take on virtually anything life dished out. It had always worked, until the cancer.

I found a large envelope in Lyse's desk and stuffed all the papers into it. Then I laid it neatly on the desk next to the calendar.

Yanking the Dust Buster out of its holster in the corner of the room, I darted into the bathroom, and vacuumed behind the toilet for any stray hairs. Then I did the entire bathroom floor, bent over, but I moved gracefully across each marble tile. I swept into each corner and under the cabinets—a morning dance I never missed. I took a quick peek under the toilet seat. Clean. Spatter-free. *Good.* I exhaled.

Before heading downstairs, I reached for the Windex under the cabinet, and soaked a paper towel. Then I wiped each bathroom countertop with forcefulness to erase any traces of hair spray, body cream, or stray eyebrow hairs.

My heart rate was up and I was breathing quickly, through my mouth. Checking my hair and makeup and satisfied that the house was in order, I called Molly into the bedroom where she would stay for the day. Bridie, our housekeeper, was scheduled to visit her at noon and 3:00 p.m. for walks and feedings. With a clotted Irish brogue, thick, work-worn hands and bright strawberry blond hair, Bridie had taken us under her wing, and had become our service provider, confidante, supporter, and chum. We adored her, and she us.

I blew Molly kisses, closed the bedroom door and flew down the steps to the foyer. Sprinting into the living room, I ran my hand under the couch cushion where Lyse sat, feeling for renegade crumbs. I pulled out two and flicked them into the kitchen garbage. I swooped up my coat and portfolio. A few minutes later, after shaking pieces of dirt and leaves off the car floor mat, I was accelerating onto Route 17 north. I drove quickly toward the hospital, breathing just a little easier.

The endoscopy and colonoscopy showed little, except a hiatal hernia, and some acid reflux disease. Dr. Hollander prescribed Nexium for the acid reflux and wished us luck during surgery the next day. Years later, I came to understand the negative impact of acidity in the body. A close friend, who is a holistic healer, had explained that cancer simply can't survive in an alkaline environment, and that the best way to avoid most disease, especially cancer, was to maintain a healthy alkaline/acidic balance—the more alkaline the better—in the body. There are foods that promote alkalinity in the body, like grapefruit, green, leafy vegetables, and figs. Processed food apparently is the worst and actually encourages acidity in the body. Lyse began having terrible reflux at night at about the time we believe the cancer was developing.

I sat at Lyse's bedside later as she poked at her meager supper. She turned up her nose at the chicken broth, but took a few sips of the hot tea. Her mood was positive and light, in spite of the imminent surgery.

The woman in the bed next to her was moaning. She was a cancer patient who had stomach pain and would receive her next chemotherapy in the hospital. When she groused, we rolled our eyes and shared uncomfortable grins across Lyse's meal tray.

At 6:00 p.m., I leaned over the cold, bulky bedside rail that dug into my left breast, and gave Lyse a soft, lingering kiss. Her lips were dry and beginning to crack.

"I'll be back early tomorrow morning, babe," I said, kissing her warm hand.

Smiling, she replied, "Okay, baby girl."

I slung my pocketbook and New York Times canvas tote bag over my shoulder, and turned around in the doorway to blow her a kiss. She looked small and vulnerable under the white sheets and cotton blanket.

I mouthed, "I love you," again, and walked into the hall.

The corridor brimmed with a powerful blend of food, medicine and ammonia odors. It was warm and suffocating. A lone nurse sat at the floor desk, rustling papers and digging for charts. I walked toward the elevators.

During the drive home, I felt the tears and worry, but I held them tightly in a little box until the right time. My ability to categorize all aspects of my life had always been very helpful and continued to be. I found, over the years, that creating a "container" or "bucket" for the many parts of my life helped me keep everything in order. Actually, it helped me manage the things that vexed me. I assigned a hypothetical container to each part of my life. Mentally, I affixed a label to each container. Each label had a name which I wrote in the Notes section at the back of my desk calendar—Lyse, House, Car, Health, Medical, Molly, Career, Dental, Eyes, Music, Friends, Family, and Finances. Sometimes I added new buckets if I needed them.

For the "Lyse" part of my life, I mentally deposited all worries, action items and thoughts about anything associated with her into the container labeled "Lyse." A misunderstanding with my sister? I'd mentally drop those troubles into the container labeled "Family." Future dental work for my problematic eyetooth? Thoughts of that went straight into the "Dental" container. Wanting to set up a new mutual fund at some point? The "Finances" bucket held those ideas.

Cataloging my life in this way has helped me organize and manage the overwhelming nature of life and what I needed to do to stay afloat. Throughout my forty-five years, this private ritual helped me mitigate the intensity of random, persistent and obsessive thoughts of what I needed to do—thoughts that coursed through my head at any given point in time.

I began the container custom in my early twenties. I began fretting when I was ten. After changing into my feetsy pajamas, I would pad out of my bedroom, and to the top of the stairs.

"Mom?" I'd call softly but with urgency.

I would hear her rustling in the living room below.

She'd answer, "Yes, Cher. What is it?"

I recited the day's events, making sure I told her everything. My words echoed and bounced slowly down each stair like a worn-out slinky. I knew she was listening from the armchair where she was darning socks, or mending Daddy's sweater.

"I went to the drug store and bought a green mechanical pencil with some of my allowance. I didn't cover my math workbook like they said I should. Let's do it tomorrow. I stopped at the park on the way home from school and climbed trees with Rose. Tomorrow is peanut butter and jelly day."

"Okay, Cher," she'd call up reassuringly. "Good night. Sleep tight."

Then I'd feel better, and would return to my bedroom. Once inside, I'd pad to the far window, near the closet. I would raise the sash and screen behind it. With precision, I'd bend over and shove my head outside into the cold, clear night air. I'd suck in its crispness while moving my head exactly one rotation to the left, and then one rotation to the right. The bright stars that clung to the dark velvet sky would blur a bit as I swung my head left and right again. I would recite my special prayer, the one I made up to protect all those I loved, whether I knew them or not. The prayer included all parts of life and heaven I might have worried about.

"God bless Mom and Dad, and Lis, and Deb, and all the animals in this world, and all the people, the past, the future and now, and everyone and everything and me."

It signaled the end of my day and helped me feel peaceful enough to climb into bed and finally let myself rest.

In my twenties, I found my container ritual to be somewhat effective and soothing, but it didn't completely erase the obsessive ruminations or anxiety. It only helped me to marginally manage a debilitating predicament.

When the worst of the worries attacked, I was beholden to a crushing adversary, an enemy I couldn't see—one that lurked deep within my gray matter, never sleeping, and never resting.

Often, the doubts centered around work. Anxieties about family or personal matters sometimes disguised themselves as work issues, which then became crippling points of apprehension.

I tried to will the worries away, and I tried to trick myself into letting go.

One more time. I'll excuse myself to the bathroom and spend three minutes working it through, and then return to the party, ready to focus and enjoy.

Sometimes it worked, but most times it didn't. Even sleep didn't banish my unease. It actually made it worse. I worried through my dreams and awoke unrefreshed and irritated, still thinking about the problem-at-hand. The sickening angst plastered against my mind like a soppy T-shirt on the spin cycle. It just kept going round and round, getting more stuck. Writing the worry down on a sticky note gave me temporary relief. But there were always more T-shirts in the laundry, and often, the void created by one distressing thought was quickly filled by another.

I watched my time off from work pass me by like a neighbor's slide show. Each picture reminded me of what I was unable to enjoy at the moment. That made me brood more. As each weekend approached, I grew uptight as others wound down. Two days away from the office could totally blow up the world I had so carefully created. One week away from the office would be more than enough time for everyone to gape at my blunders under the glare of those blinding fluorescent lights.

Chapter Four:
It Really is Cancer

Obsessive-Compulsive Disorder, OCD, is an anxiety disorder and is characterized by recurrent, unwanted thoughts (obsessions) and/or repetitive behaviors (compulsions). Repetitive behaviors such as hand-washing, counting, checking, or cleaning are often performed with the hope of preventing obsessive thoughts or making them go away.

National Institute of Mental Health
www.nimh.nih.gov

Wednesday, September 25, 2002

Late that afternoon, I had called Mom from Lyse's bedside to wish her a happy birthday. I told her that Lyse had cancer. Her voice was reassuring, sorrowful, and comforting. Lyse had been in surgery for close to five hours but had done well in spite of the extensive procedure.

Monique, and Jeannie, with husband, Ron, had arrived from New England early that afternoon. Before their arrival, I had gone out to the car for a nap. I dozed fitfully and got up feeling very fatigued, and hazy. After I brought the seat back to an upright position, and felt satisfied that it was aligned with the passenger seat, I locked the car and walked back toward the hospital. I saw their car pull into the parking lot. Ron was driving, as he always did. I smiled and waved with all of the pluck I could muster and walked, heavy-legged, to meet them.

Monique gave me a warm and welcoming hug. She was the earth-mother, a cooing presence everyone was grateful for. Short of stature and fleshly, she represented softness and comfort—a way station along the formidable road of life. Ron embraced me shyly, but affectionately. Jeannine's gaze was piercing and questioning. I reached out and hugged her politely.

Lowering her strawberry-blonde head and with her eyes boring downward, she muttered, "Well, we've got our hands full, don't we?"

Her alluring French-Canadian lilt did little to disguise the anger and angst she seethed. I was the logical scapegoat—the one who last saw her baby sister—the one who had all the information. I was overcome with the weight of fixing this, making it right for Lyse, and making it right for her sorrow-stricken sisters.

Did Jeannine think I had caused Lyse to get sick?

Jeannine was the essence of good health. Her years in nursing had given her a leg up on how to sustain good health and prevent disease through vitamins and simple home remedies. Years of beholding the ravages of disease had spooked her. So, she compensated through meticulous self-care. Wiry and chipper, she exuded vigor through bright eyes and favorable pallor. Focused on good nutrition in every meal, she cooked with only the freshest ingredients—many of them fruits and vegetables from her own little garden behind the house in Attleboro, Massachusetts. It wasn't unusual for Jeannine to give us overflowing bags of beefsteak tomatoes, bright red, plump and laden with juice. Ron agreed, for the most part, to her strict meal plan, but it also wasn't uncommon for him to venture out alone for a burger and beer when a craving struck.

I escorted the nerve-jangled trio back to the hospital and we headed to the cafeteria. They ordered coffee and bagels and I had a diet Coke, welcoming the caffeine in spite of my tight insides.

I methodically and calmly updated them on the doctors, the tests, and the plan for the day. It was close to 2:00 p.m. Lyse would soon be in surgery.

We waited for about five hours. Ron had gone out to the car for a nap. He checked on us intermittently during the afternoon. Monique, Jeannine and I sat in the family waiting room. We dozed, read, and exchanged terse snippets of dialogue.

"The longer she's in there, the better her chances," Jeannine blurted out tensely.

"So that's a good thing, then?" I replied gently.

"Oh, yes," Monique jumped in, with brightness in her voice. "They brought Georgette out after a half hour. They opened her, saw they couldn't do anything, and then closed her back up."

Plus, that was fourteen years ago—the stone age for cancer treatment.

Georgette had been fourteen years Lyse's senior but they were close. The siblings had enjoyed perching on the rocks at the water in Providence, Rhode Island, sucking down little neck clams and cold glasses of beer. Georgette had been a nurse also, and had worked with Jeannine for many years at the Women and Infants' Hospital in Providence.

"Every hour the clock goes by means they're cleaning her out and making some progress," Jeannine continued, her face stiff with worry.

"Hmmm…that's really good, then," I replied with enthusiasm. "In that case, we'll be grateful for every hour the clock turns."

We sat quietly, listening to the announcements and pages for doctors and waiting family members. The TV droned in the background—occasional laughter and audience applause pierced the monotony. Other people who were waiting looked as we did. Some napped, heads slung over the maroon fabric chairs, some read, and anxiously looked up in-between pages. People talked in hushed tones, as if being too vocal might interfere with the critical work of the surgeons.

I'm so worried about Lyse I can't even worry about work. Everything I have to worry about at work is written down on my calendar and Post-it notes. It's all written down. Don't worry. I can't worry. I can't worry.

I reached into my New York Times bag for my bottle of aspirin. My headache was the kind that would only get worse if I didn't take something immediately. I swallowed three Anacins with a swig of my diet Coke. I closed my eyes and their sting lessened a bit.

Monique returned from the chapel and told us how peaceful it was. She said she prayed and asked the lord to help all of us right now, to help Lyse be courageous and strong. She told us she prayed the rosary and asked if I would like to do the same.

The waiting room was quiet. Doctors and nurses breezed down the corridor, with their white coattails flying out behind them like kites.

"No, thank you," I responded quietly. "I'm not Catholic, but I've been praying all along and I guess the good lord will hear all of us, no matter how we talk to him."

Monique smiled and I asked to see her rosary. The mauve beads were warm and smooth in my hand. I was briefly comforted.

At 4:55 p.m., a blaring pager announcement sliced the silence. It instructed all family members to go to the nighttime waiting area down the hall on the right. About nine of us grumbled in unison. Then we straggled wearily into a room that was cold and uninviting. Scuffed linoleum flooring intersected with a faded and stained tan carpet further inside the room. Aluminum chairs scraped the floor as people got settled.

The others, with whom we had bonded a little during the day, showed telltale signs of their day of waiting—dark circles under dull eyes, Styrofoam cups in which coffee had long ago turned tepid, half-eaten candy bars, and clothing that had evolved into disheveled and crumpled messes.

As I used the ladies room—stress diarrhea continued to plague me—I heard a male voice, possibly that of Dr. Huss, and then Monique talking to Jeannine.

Oh my god! Crap!

"Wait. Let me get Cheryl. She's in the ladies room. Don't start without her," I heard Monique's muffled and panicky voice through the thick, wooden lavatory door.

Monique rapped loudly and told me Dr. Huss was waiting to give us the report.

Oh, my god. The minute he comes out of surgery, I'm in here having a poop attack! Of course. Ugh!

I clenched my teeth and held in what I hadn't finished. *It can wait.* I was shaking and my heart raced. I jammed down the toilet handle, and stumbled out to the waiting room. The right side of my sage Eddie Bauer sweater was hiked up over my right hip, and tangled in my T-shirt.

Dr. Huss stood there in his scrubs holding a notepad. He looked unruffled but somewhat perplexed.

"Everything went well," he relayed softly. "She's in recovery right now, doing well. We removed the ovaries and they were biopsied. Cancer was found in the left ovary. It was peculiar that her ovaries were small, very small, and that is unusual for ovaries that are cancerous."

I felt that I might just vomit, and I heard a loud buzzing inside my head. I pinched myself hard with my fingernails to counteract the nausea. *Ouch!* I pinched again. For a moment, I didn't hear Dr. Huss's voice but I saw his lips moving. My heart rammed against my chest. I felt its beat in the back of my throat. My breathing was tight and labored.

"We removed the malignant fluid in Lyse's peritoneum," he continued matter-of-factly.

"We also performed a total hysterectomy. We debulked as much of the malignant tissue as we could, removing most of it, but there are microscopic seedings that remain in the diaphragm. These are what we hope to target with chemotherapy. I'm sorry I don't have better news. Lyse will be ready to see the family in a couple of hours, once she is more awake."

Dr. Huss looked very tired, but boyish, despite his advanced years. We clung to his monologue. The three of us hung on to every word, and hoped

The Dust Busting Chronicles

that the longer he talked he would speak of a total cure, a procedure that would somehow restore Lyse's health.

The operative report would later read:

Post Operative Diagnosis: Frozen section, ovarian cancer, primary with metastatic disease to the peritoneum, omentum and diaphragm in the form of small seedings and infiltration of the omentum in the form of nodular thickenings, small fibroid on the uterus, normal uterus.

After Dr. Huss left, we stood and looked at each other with sallow and defeated faces. We repeated much of what he had relayed, and built upon it, trying to find the notches on which we could rest some hope—like a skilled rock climber might do in reaching for a solid toe-hold.

"Sounds like they removed most of the cancer. That's very good," Jeannine said with conviction.

"It seems possible that the chemotherapy can get rid of the few seedings that are left," I offered with a faux calmness. "At least she's being given the chance to fight it. Sounds like Dr. Huss and Dr. Gennaoui think she has a chance if they're at least talking about chemotherapy," I continued, feeling somewhat hopeful and invigorated.

Ron returned from outside and Jeannine updated him. He shook his head over and over again, dejectedly.

"Why don't we go get something to eat while Lyse is still in recovery?" Jeannine suggested. "We could all use a break by now."

Ron suggested Applebee's. It was right down the road from the hospital. I sank into the soft leather seat of Ron and Jeannine's Acura, and felt my overwrought muscles relax slightly. I took a deep breath and closed my eyes.

I don't remember what I ate for dinner that night. Maybe it was the rib eye special. It may have come with a baked potato. I may have had a glass of wine. I may have been hungry, or not. All I know now, years later, is that I'll never be able to eat another meal at the chain with the fruit in its name.

❧

We returned to the hospital around 7:00 p.m. Lyse looked good, considering her time in surgery. Jeannine kept commenting on Lyse's plump, rosy lips. It was a comical pause in the gravity of the moment and it felt good to laugh.

She was also very encouraged by Lyse's pallor and general responsiveness. We spoke with Lyse briefly about the outcome of surgery and she took it in good stride, without alarm, as I knew she would.

Lyse never really overreacted to anything. She carried an even temper and took most things in stride. She became angry, when she needed to. Like the night my flight from Chicago arrived at Newark Int'l Airport at 1:00 a.m. and my waiting car took another customer because I was late.

She gave the surprised dispatcher a good tongue-lashing, and made him culpable for my well-being and safety in that desolate and cavernous baggage zone.

The family trio stayed at the Hilton Hotel down the street and returned to see Lyse the next morning before heading back to Massachusetts.

I'm so grateful they didn't ask to stay with me. There would be more cleaning to do. Oh my god. I would freak out for sure. The bathroom would be the worst. I'm so grateful. I'm so glad about it that I can even deal with the guilt about not asking them.

Ron would drive Jeannine back to the hospital a few days later when Lyse was discharged. I kissed Lyse. I told her how well she had done, and that I was really proud of her.

"We're going to get through this together, babe," I said optimistically. "I'll be right next to you every step of the way," I offered softly, kissing her forehead and smiling.

She looked at me with tears in her eyes—melancholy emanated from her every pore. She smiled in spite of it and I gave her another peck on the cheek. Her eyes were heavy and she was ready for sleep again.

"I love you, baby," I whispered.

"I love you, too," she replied with a sigh, as her gentle, brown eyes closed.

I hugged Jeannie, Ron and Monique and headed past the eerily quiet nurse's station, toward the elevator. A few minutes later, as Manhattan's public radio station, NPR, launched its 10:00 p.m. news, I drove down Route 17 south toward home.

I pulled into the driveway a half-hour later, and I noticed the soft lights behind the drapes and blinds of the neighbors' buttoned-up homes. The adrenaline was still coursing through my veins but I was calmed somewhat as I glanced in the rearview mirror at Leo and Camille's cozy house across the street. I gathered my bags and headed upstairs, loudly calling to Molly so she could hear me through the closed bedroom door.

My first stop was the kitchen. I continued talking to Molly as I scanned the counters, floor and sink to see what crumbs or streaks Bridie had left from her visit with Molly that afternoon. I soaked a paper towel with Windex, bent down and wiped the floor next to the sink, counter and stove. My heart pounded.

Once I get this done, I can relax.

A few crumbs and a piece of Molly's wet food showed up on the paper towel, so I turned it over and wiped the floor again.

Jeez. Why is there stuff on the floor?

I ripped a clean paper towel, sprayed Windex on the counter next to the sink, and wiped it vigorously. Before tossing it, I wiped down the handles on the faucet, microwave and refrigerator door.

"Coming, Mols, coming, sweetie," I called. "Hang on, baby."

My voice cracked with fatigue. My muscles were sucked dry of strength and energy. I pushed to finish wiping down the countertop. I raced upstairs and opened the door to the bedroom. Molly bounded into my arms. She was full of kisses and love, and shook with happiness to see me. I hugged and kissed her. Then I rubbed her belly and drew in her sweet smell.

The phone rang.

Damn! Why are people bothering me?

It was Camille.

"How did everything go today with the surgery?" she asked, her cheerful voice so bright I squinted.

I gave her a brief rundown, and she offered to bring me a plate for dinner the next day. I thanked her for calling and then hung up.

Our neighbors are so caring. We're so lucky. But I'm so angry that our lives are all screwed up and I have to keep talking about it to the neighbors who keep asking. Why don't they get it? Don't they see how intrusive and exhausting it is for me?

After I took Molly out and gave her a treat, I yanked the Dust Buster out of its holster in the powder room on the first floor, anxious to complete my cleaning. I walked downstairs to the basement and worked my way up the steps, sucking up pieces of grass and dirt from each corner. It was satisfying to hear the soft clink of granules being sucked into the vacuum.

How does all this gunk end up on the floor? There's more inside our house than on the front lawn. It's ridiculous!

I continued up the steps. The adrenaline gave new zing to my legs.

A small smile broke my scowl. I remembered dust busting the crumbs on Lyse's chest after she enjoyed a Pepperidge Farm Milano cookie on the couch last month. She laughed, and then so did I when I realized the absurdity of what I was doing. What I remember now is the unconditional love we shared in that moment.

I swiped the vacuum under the edge of the mauve Oriental rug in the foyer, and did the same around the sides of the blue wool runner that separated the dining room and the kitchen. I did a once-over of the kitchen floor, and spent a few seconds under the sage and plum throw rug at the sink.

I feel better. Now, my drink. My brandy. In bed.

I poured a shot-and-a-half of Benedictine and Brandy—B&B, our favorite sweet and biting nightcap—into a Waterford crystal four ounce snifter. The bright amber colored liquid emitted a luscious perfume—a flower pool into which I could dump the heartaches of my day. After taking a deep breath, I turned off the lights, and climbed the steps slowly. I cradled the cool, angular glass in my palm. I undressed, gulped 2 mg of my Xanax, and walked quietly toward the soft comfort of our bed. The tears I held back earlier in the day heaved at the back of my leaden eyes. They came easy, as did my sleep.

Chapter Five:
Finding Our Way

I have always been able to compensate for my OCD, knowing that it was my way of coming out on top of anything life threw my way. But the cancer was something way bigger than anything I could do with Windex and a Dust Buster.

In the beginning of our relationship, it wasn't unusual for Lyse and me to spend an entire Sunday afternoon lazing on the living room floor of my small apartment, gazing at the fall foliage through the charming casement windows. Celine Dion, Enya, Ella Fitzgerald and Schumann serenaded us through those dreamy afternoons. We cuddled, snoozed and lost ourselves in our other-world, temporarily suspended in time with affection and attention richly lavished on each other. We'd order in Chinese food—chicken with snow peas and spare ribs—and work our way through a bottle of Chardonnay. I cooked also, easy meals that didn't tax my narrow culinary skill set. We enjoyed instant rice and beans, linguine with pasta sauce from a jar, and chicken tenders I sprinkled with lemon pepper and tossed in the microwave. Our budding love transformed those elementary meals into flavorful banquets.

I was falling in love. No, I was in love. I was feeling all of it. Love, love and more love. I wanted to offer up all of myself to this fifty-five-year-old woman with the beautiful smile and silver hair. I held nothing back and yielded my body to her abundant and welcoming flesh. Loving someone. In love with someone. Two very different things, I discovered, during my precious eight years with Lyse.

On our first date at Barnes & Noble, on May 3, 1996, I described my antique BMW motorcycle, and told her that "antique" in the cycling world meant that a bike was at least twenty-five years old. I was uncertain of her age at that time, so she told me, with a nervous smile, that she was at least "two antiques old." I really didn't think she was much younger than that, given her silver hair, so I wasn't completely surprised. She was clearly uncomfortable though, and I later found out that she worried about the "robbing the cradle" thing.

Baby, if you're the hottie robbing cradles, let me turn off the ADT and wait on the front porch.

It took her at least two years before she could kind of forget about the age difference. I think what worried her most was the intuitive feeling that I would get "the short end of the stick." What worried me most was my premonition that we would only have a short time together. We had both been right.

Monday, September 30, 2002

Lyse was being discharged today. Ron and Monique left this morning to go back to New England. Jeannine and I waited patiently while Lyse's discharge instructions were prepared. Drs. Huss and Gennaoui saw Lyse earlier this morning and gave her the "all clear."

Late last week, Dr. Huss referred Lyse to Dr. Sushil Bhardwaj (bod-wash), Director of Oncology at the hospital. This past Friday, Dr. Bhardwaj met with us in Lyse's room for a consultation. He wore a dark, expensive suit, crisp cotton shirt, and a lustrous lavender tie. His demeanor was pleasant and he radiated all of the confidence one would expect from a seemingly successful physician. He smiled broadly, displaying glossy teeth against his dark skin.

At first glance, he appeared the kind of doctor we needed, wanted, hoped for—someone very caring, gentle, approachable, and highly-skilled. After the initial exchange, though, he abruptly puffed up and feathers sprung forth. He emphatically told us about his state-of-the-art cancer center, made possible by very generous donations from local benefactors. For several long minutes, he reeled off qualifications and statistics that caused my eyes to dull. Lyse's eyes had already glazed over. She looked pale and worn out.

In choppy English, he continued, "So, you'll come by for a tour this week, and we'll get you all set up for treatment?"

"We haven't yet chosen an oncologist and want to look at all the options we have before making a decision," Lyse explained quietly, yet tenaciously.

Brows knitted and smile fading, he replied, "Well, I think you'll find that our services here are the very best. You can look at Sloan-Kettering, Hackensack, or wherever you want, but we have top care here and you may be disappointed elsewhere. All the others are not always what you think they are."

"Thank you, doctor, for your time today," Lyse offered, smiling. "We appreciate you meeting with us and we'll be in touch if we decide to move forward with you."

Realizing his done deal wasn't done, Dr. Bhardwaj (hog wash) shook our hands quickly and hurtled from the room, with his white coat billowing behind him, propelling him away from us like a sail.

Before Lyse could go home, she needed to prove she could climb a flight of stairs by herself. A young physical therapist told her how to walk and climb steps while supporting her abdomen. She shuffled over to the set of trial stairs on the other side of the hallway and tackled them slowly, but successfully.

"I never thought I'd be learning to walk again at this age," Lyse told the therapist, a smile brightening her face briefly.

I was encouraged by her spirit.

Thirty minutes later, the three of us, and an aide who pushed Lyse's wheelchair, made our way downstairs. I got the car and met everyone outside the hospital lobby. I had already loaded Lyse's things—a white, plastic "Patient Belongings" bag and her overnight bag—into the trunk. The Patient Belongings bag saddened me. When it comes right down to matters of crisis or illness, we are all stripped of our material support system and left with just the clothes on our backs, and perhaps a pair of eyeglasses. We then grow humbled—transformed into indigent and vulnerable little creatures—fully reliant on the kindness and goodness of those willing to fend for us in our time of need.

Jeannine and the sinewy young, black, male aide supported Lyse on each side as she slowly rolled herself into the front seat. Groaning from fatigue, she closed her eyes and rested briefly. Her cheeks were ashen.

We arrived home and Lyse reluctantly unfurled herself from the car seat. After we walked with her up the short driveway, she slowly climbed the cement stairs up to the front door. Jeannine was on her left side, her hand grasped the railing on the right, and I cradled her bottom from behind. We did the same for the eight steps up to the dining room from the foyer, and the two sets of seven steps from the dining room to the second floor.

She's already lost a couple of pounds. Her pants are loose and her hiney has lost some of its sexy roundness. Hmmm.

I was distracted and worried by this thought.

After Lyse settled into bed, I quickly grabbed my bag and keys. I told Lyse and Jeannine that I was going to CVS to pick up Lyse's medication. She'd been prescribed Prevacid, for the acid reflux, and acetaminophen with codeine for the pain. She might have needed the meds right away so I didn't want to wait. The trip to the pharmacy was about a half-mile. I enjoyed the warmth of the sun streaming through the windows. It softened the sharp edges of my muscles, which were angular with tension. My eyes grew heavy in the snug warmth of the cabin.

Once home, I ran the bag of pills upstairs, and then began to feverishly compile Lyse's papers for Sloan-Kettering. I'd made an appointment for Lyse at the Center's Rockefeller Outpatient Pavilion, 160 E. 53rd Street, Manhattan. We had a consultation scheduled with Dr. Sybil Anderson on Tuesday, October 8, at 1:00 p.m. I was burdened to see that Lyse received only the finest medical care. We needed to be seen by the experts at Sloan-Kettering to make sure we were taking advantage of the latest and finest treatment options. Only the best for Lyse.

Memorial Sloan-Kettering Cancer Center has provided care for over a century, and is a champion in the cancer world. As depicted on its web site, *www.mskcs.org*, the center is "the oldest and largest private cancer center in the world." The center "promotes physicians and scientists working closely together to develop and implement state-of-the-art prevention, therapies and cures."

Tracy Agar, from registration, instructed me to fax specific medical documents so she could forward them to Dr. Anderson for review, before we met with her. These included the following: hospital release, operative report, pathology report, CT scan report, discharge summary, history and physical report, consultative report, and lab reports.

I had requested these documents from Good Samaritan's Records Department but found the process of obtaining them a little tricky. After I completed a couple of request forms, showed the clerk Lyse's power of attorney, and waited for two days, I was able to pick them up.

While Jeannine prepared a light lunch for Lyse—a soft boiled egg on toast, and a cup of tea, which Lyse liked black with two sugars—I prepared my fax cover sheet for Tracy. There were twenty-two sheets, including the cover page.

OK. Everything's fine. Don't worry. OK. All I have to do now is fax this package to Tracy, and then maybe I can take a nap.

My breathing was fast and uneven. I could hear my heart in my ears. Flying into the spare bedroom/office with the pile of papers, I turned on the fax machine, plugged in the phone cord, and dialed Sloan-Kettering's number.

The machine connected. Page one wasn't being pulled through the feeder. Unfamiliar machine noises screeched at me through the fax.

"If you'd like to make a call, please hang up and dial again," the operator instructed me.

"What are you talking about, lady?" I hissed at the machine.

My stomach churned and I felt acid secreting into my gurgling belly. I checked the phone line connection and the power cord. They all looked good. I hit cancel and tried again. Same thing.

Oh my god. What is wrong with this piece of crap? I don't believe this!

The afternoon sun streamed into the window, and bathed the desk, the bed and me in sultry light. It quickly warmed the room and caused a light sweat to form on my forehead and upper lip. Strands of hair from my braid came loose and I angrily wiped them away. I ripped off my sweater and enjoyed a brief coolness that found its way onto my torso, damp under my T-shirt.

I heard Jeannine and Lyse talking quietly, even giggling now and again, sharing family stories and bits of news. Lyse's tone of voice implied easy, enjoyable banter, and projected a calmness I had not heard in a few days. I was grateful Jeannine was with us.

I yanked the phone cord out of the fax machine, plugged it into the phone, and lifted the receiver to see if the phone was working. Furiously, I dialed Sloan-Kettering's number and heard ringing. Then, over the ringing, the screech of a fax machine as it tried to make a connection.

Tracy Agar answered the phone but she sounded like she was in a tunnel. The fax machine had stopped screeching but the phone line continued to ring while Tracy and I spoke. A trickle of perspiration ran between my breasts.

"Tracy, this is Cheryl Cushine, for Lyse St. Denis. I'm trying to fax Lyse's medical records to you but I'm having trouble with my fax machine, as you can hear."

The ringing had stopped but my voice, and everything I said, echoed right back at me. It was as if the fax and phone line were both carrying my call.

Maybe this is how a psychotic feels—voices and strange noises all out of sequence, an unpredictable barrage of nonsensical sounds.

Just then, I started laughing, and I sputtered almost, as gobs of silliness spurted out of my mouth. I tried to stop, but I suddenly felt featherbrained and muddle-headed.

Choking down the peals of giddiness to maintain some semblance of professionalism, I eked out, "Why don't I find another fax machine—my neighbor should have one—and I'll have the documents to you later this afternoon."

Spurt. Giggle. Spurt.

Tracy was somewhat amused by the ridiculous electronic snafu, and wished me luck with the phone.

I called Bell Atlantic service to schedule a repair for the phone line. Then, I walked into the master bedroom to share my laughable misfortune with Lyse and Jeannine, holding my sides while shrieking and snorting. We enjoyed the folly.

∽

When I was thirteen, my parents divorced and Mom, my sisters Lisa and Deb, and I moved from Pennington, New Jersey to Ventnor Heights, New Jersey. Ventnor is a suburb of Atlantic City and the Heights sits west of town. When we moved in, Mom bought a shag area rug for my room. It was purple—my favorite color—and inexpensive. It covered about three-quarters of my bedroom.

Every Saturday I dusted my room, and vacuumed the rug. I'd avoid walking on the rug, for fear of squashing the long, vertical fibers and ruining the perfectly coiffed piece. I took great pains to walk around the rug, hopping into bed from the foot of it, and reaching into my dresser drawers with my feet planted at a forty-five degree angle from the rest of me, on the wooden part of the floor.

As long as the purple rug retained its just brushed look, I felt good, and was calm inside—less fretful. By about Tuesday, smashed areas of a six-and-one-half shoe size emerged. I tried perking up the fibers with my hand, even using my hairbrush, to get it back to the just-vacuumed look.

Clean floors, shiny toilets, and spot-free counters lessen my anxiety around stressful situations. The amount of control I feel I have over a stressful event is directly proportional to the volume of cleaning and organizing I can accomplish.

❧

After the fax machine debacle, I called Leo next door and asked if I could use his fax machine. He told me to come right over.

"How's Lyse?" he asked with furrowed brow.

A semi-retired executive, his basement office boasted a plush, rust colored leather sofa and recliner, dark, heavy, wooden computer desk and bookshelves, widescreen television, sound system, printer/fax/scanner, and an oversized busy Oriental rug. It was cozy in his office and I was envious of the routine day he appeared to be having.

"She's doing all right, Leo," I replied, sighing more loudly than I expected.

He towered above me—a tall, big man of Irish heritage, he had thick silver hair which fell onto his forehead. I felt small and vulnerable. The weight of Lyse's illness seemed even heavier as I stood in front of my burly, confident neighbor. I wanted to flop onto his couch and sleep for a couple of hours.

"At least she's home from the hospital now and her sister Jeannine is caring for her round the clock," I continued, trying to muster enough energy to at least project my voice up to where his ears were. "She'll be starting chemo soon and we're optimistic that she has a decent fighting chance."

He looked really worried, and just shook his head. He and Lyse had worked on the board of the townhouse association for two years. He was very fond of her. They appreciated each other's clever wit and thought alike when it came to resolving community issues.

"Well, that's good," he replied. "We're so worried about her, and you. I just don't understand how something like this happens to a woman like Lyse."

Leo turned on his fax machine. He looked at the package for Sloan-Kettering and said we should number each page. He did that for me. Twenty-five minutes later, I was back home. Sloan-Kettering had Lyse's records.

As I headed upstairs to check on Lyse and take a nap, I heard something. Music. A piano. Singing. It was coming through the wall in the living room—the wall with the couch. A woman was singing, with a piano accompaniment.

It's our Korean neighbor next door! Oh my god! It's like she's in our living room!

My stomach lurched and felt sour. My heart pounded in my eardrums as my anger rose.

Our fair-skinned, round-faced neighbor was about forty-three years old and lived with her eight-year-old daughter. According to Leo, Mr. Kim, the owner of the townhouse, was renting the unit to her for six months while she promoted her career as a pop singer, touring clubs in the New York/New Jersey Korean community. As a rule of thumb, Mr. Kim only rented to Koreans, as Leo relayed it.

It's like she waited until Lyse came home from the hospital to start practicing! I can't believe this! There's no way I can stand this noise coming into our house! Lyse is trying to recuperate and needs to rest. This is totally unacceptable! Crap!

I stomped downstairs to the front door, slipped into my clogs, and marched right over to her house. I was breathing heavily, and I gasped for air. My fatigue was replaced by fury. Pressing hard for good measure, I rang the bell three times.

I can hear the music through her own front door! This is ridiculous! She can't even hear the doorbell over her own racket!

After several more rings of the bell, she finally came to the door. She wore black jeans and a bright purple cashmere sweater. An ugly gold and purple stone pin sat below her left shoulder. Her graying hair was tossed up on top of her head in a loose bun. She was wearing no makeup and I almost didn't recognize her.

"Hi," I said with no smile. I offered no pleasantries. "Lyse is recuperating from major surgery," I blurted out, pointing to our house, in case she needed reminding which one was ours. My composed corporate demeanor was nowhere to be found. "We can hear your piano and singing right through our living room wall."

My voice was steady and strong, as was my eye contact with her. My insides were spasming from the troubles of the day.

"I so sorry about Lyse, but I must sing during day for concert at night. I no help piano," she replied, the pitch of her voice rising slightly.

She motioned me inside so I could see that the piano was not close to the wall. Rather, it was a couple of feet from it.

"I play with pedal to make less noise," she offered.

The damper pedal would have helped a bit, but I suspected the sound would still travel.

"Can you move the piano to the other wall?" I asked, my face hot and heart racing. "The sound is really very loud! Lyse can't rest with the noise!"

"I see maybe we move piano. I don't know but try," she said, perturbed, with her voice rising.

"Please see what you can do, then," I replied. I walked toward the front door. "Thank you," I said tersely, turning to leave.

On my way back to the house, Leo called to me as he crossed the street. I told him what had happened and he agreed to talk with our neighbor on our behalf. Leo was a true diplomat—a genteel, yet firm man of the highest integrity, and a skilled consensus builder. I was grateful for his intervention.

Other than a bit of quiet tinkling from the piano later that afternoon, we never heard the music again.

Tuesday, October 1, 2002

Ding dong, ding dong. The doorbell started ringing today and continued all week. Each time I answered it, there was a new delivery person waiting, with full arms and a smile. Every time it jingled, Molly's shrieky bark pierced the quiet of the house and echoed up to the bedroom where Lyse was napping, reading or watching old movies.

A basket from Tenafly's Sunshine Club arrived first. Three jumbo grapefruit sat atop a pile of goodies in a wicker basket that was wrapped in yellow cellophane. Peering through the crinkly paper, I saw water crackers, biscuits, imported chocolates, hot chocolate, cheese, pears and gourmet nuts. The card, stapled to the outside, read: "Dear Lyse, We're thinking of you and miss you. Hurry back! Regards, The Tenafly Middle School Teachers." Molly was nudging me, so I let her sniff the cumbersome basket, and then I took it upstairs to show Lyse. She had been napping but awakened when she heard my footsteps.

Smiling, and groggy, she eyed the basket and said, "Wow. That's really nice."

I told her I was going to put the goodies away, and then headed back downstairs. *Ding dong. Ding dong. Ding dong.* I looked down to the driveway from the kitchen where I had just started unpacking the Sunshine basket. A truck from Wine and Roses florist in New Milford had just pulled up. Molly raced to the top of the steps and began to yip while scampering back and forth on the landing.

The delivery woman handed me a magnificent bouquet of lilies, snapdragons, mums and roses that sprang out of a large, dark green clay vase. It was very heavy. I carried it up to the living room and placed it near the fireplace. The gift was from Judy, Joan, Etta and Diane, four of Lyse's colleagues from the middle school. Judy and Lyse had been friends and coworkers for over twenty years and were very close.

Ding dong. Ding dong. A van was pulling up now. More barking from Molly while I raced down to the front door. The driver was walking up the steps with a cookie bouquet.

Oh my god. Enough with the food deliveries already. How are we going to eat all of this? Where am I going to put it?

I smiled politely and thanked the driver. My teeth were clenched. My jaw was sore. Wearily, I climbed the steps to the bedroom to show Lyse the gift. She opened the card. It was from Bridie and her daughter, Tara, who also taught at the middle school. A year before, Lyse had helped Tara navigate the interview process, and offered a recommendation on her behalf.

The cookies were gigantic—at least four inches in diameter. They were all decorated like flowers, in bright colors with icing and candy pieces. Green

Easter basket straw covered the bottom of the basket and the cookies were on wooden sticks at least seven inches tall.

Well, at least Lyse won't lose any weight if she eats these.

Jeannine and Lyse smiled at the cute arrangement. Lyse was clearly pleased at the outpouring of well-wishers.

I flew back downstairs to unpack all the baskets and put the food away. Molly raced after me, and gasped from the excitement.

Cheese and fruit in the fridge. Nuts and crackers in the pantry. Cookies off the sticks. Freeze half of them and keep the other half in Tupperware in the pantry. Cookie basket in the garbage. Crumbs off the counter. Done.

The obsessions and/or compulsions are great enough to cause significant distress in [their] employment, schoolwork, or personal and social relationships.

www.athealth.com

Ding dong. Ding dong.

Crap. Who now? Oh my god. Another delivery? I can't believe this.

I felt my jaw tighten again. A van from Oradell Florist was in the driveway. I raced down the steps and opened the front door. The smiling, middle-aged delivery woman handed me a mid-sized bouquet of pink roses, carnations, baby's breath and heather, snug in a chunky glass vase. I thanked her, closed the door, and raced up the three flights of stairs to the bedroom to present the flowers to Lyse. On my way up, I checked the card. The arrangement was from Monique and her husband, Bob.

Jeannine was sponge-bathing her sister. She had filled up the unused pink vomit bucket from the hospital with warm, soapy water and was gently swabbing the area around the incision with a washcloth.

Is she spilling any water on the bed? The floor?

A messy hodgepodge of tissues, books, the TV remote, and a small bowl of saltines sat on the nightstand. I was flustered and distracted by the chaos on Lyse's side of the bed.

Some of the most prevalent compulsions are: repeated checking of doors, locks, electrical appliances, or light switches, frequent cleaning of hands or clothes, strict attempts to keep various, personal items in careful order, and mental activities that are repetitious, such as counting or praying.

www.athealth.com

"Sweetie, this bouquet is from Monique and Bob. How about we leave this one up here for you to enjoy?" I said gently. "I've put the other arrangements in the living room so it doesn't get too cluttered up here," I continued.

"Sure, that will be fine," Lyse replied drowsily.

She looked pale and uncomfortable. Jeannine was making sure that she got enough pain medication. Drawing on her nursing prowess, she was able to interpret Lyse's complaints of "discomfort" as pain, and gave her the right amount of the narcotic analgesic.

Lyse looked over at me and asked, "Are you doing OK, babe?" Her eyes showed concern for me in spite of her own discomfort. "I know it's a lot right now."

"Uh huh," I replied with a smile and lingering gaze. "You just rest and take care of yourself, babe."

I mouthed, "I love you," and she did the same, smiling wanly.

"Everyone is really thinking about you, Lyse," Jeannine piped up cheerily. "It's so nice of them."

"I know," Lyse responded. "I'm blessed to have such caring friends."

I was pleased that friends and coworkers had rallied around her, and were giving her support and attention. Her humbleness and modesty were like a magnet for some. They sensed her quiet strength, her integrity and inner peace. They were curious about her inner sanctity. They were drawn to it.

Tuesday, October 8, 2002

We made our way into Manhattan for our appointment with Dr. Sybil Anderson. Cathy and Joanne were with us. I didn't want the extra stress of driving into the city and trying to park, so I hired a car for the trip.

Cathy and I had been friends for eighteen years—she was my oldest and dearest friend—and her partner, Joanne, was Molly's vet. The four of us had developed a solid and harmonious friendship, centered around long, passionate talks over wine and play dates with our Yorkies. Their four boys, Nicholas, Toby, Simon and Sebastian (Sebby) were Molly's half-brothers. Some of my happiest memories were of watching the five "kids" play, then conk out on the dog beds in front of the fireplace.

Sloan-Kettering's 53rd Street location covered eleven floors and offered outpatient radiation and chemotherapy services, in addition to various clinics such as gynecology and cardiology. We found our way up to the sixth floor to complete the paperwork for registration and patient financial services. Cathy and Joanne had packed snacks for us—carrots, nuts, granola bars, and iced tea—which we munched on while waiting for our one o'clock consultation.

Patients and their families lounged on comfortable couches and armchairs. Fruit juice and lemon water were available in the corner of the room. The rugs were thick and colorful. Bright, heavy drapes and soothing wall color created a warm ambiance.

"Lyse St. Denis?" a young man in a white lab coat asked, walking toward us.

"Yes, that's me," Lyse replied and stood up to shake his hand.

"I'm Chris Autry. Nice to meet you. I work with Dr. Anderson. I'm going to take your history, and then Dr. Anderson will be in to meet with you."

Chris was a Fellow at the center. His demeanor was warm, and polished. I had already prepared a list of bullet points I wanted to discuss: chemotherapy treatment plan, treatment drugs and side effects, caregiver support anticipated, and chemotherapy "do's and don'ts." Cathy had also prepared a list of concerns she wanted to make sure were addressed. Cathy and Joanne were our extra pair of eyes and ears—the people who could be more objective than we could ever be. We would come to find their emotional support invaluable.

The volume of information we were given by so many sources was such that Cathy and Joanne's ability to process it and ask their own sets of questions insured that we didn't miss a thing.

We were taken to a small exam room where Chris asked questions about Lyse's symptoms, surgery, diagnosis, and family background. Several minutes later, a young, energetic, tall, thin black woman breezed into the room. She was not wearing a lab coat.

"Lyse?" she asked, extending her hand to Lyse, who was sitting on the exam table. "I'm Dr. Anderson."

I was concerned that we were not meeting with a doctor who was a little more seasoned, but considered she had to be good if she practiced here.

Dr. Anderson drew the curtain around the table and examined Lyse. She then reviewed Chris's notes and glanced at Lyse's medical records.

"So, you haven't been feeling very well, huh?" Dr. Anderson asked Lyse.

"Thing is, I've always been really healthy, except for the cancer!" Lyse replied, and we all laughed.

The doctor told us that the standard protocol, for the stage of disease Lyse had, was debulking surgery first, and then chemotherapy—six rounds of Carboplatin and Taxol three weeks apart. Then, depending upon the results of that, they would infuse medication directly into the peritoneal cavity via a port. A laparoscope would be used to monitor and gauge the status of the peritoneal chemotherapy.

She went on to say that the peritoneal treatment was a relatively new procedure with little to no clinical data available. It had been offered by the center on a trial basis since 1999, with good results.

Later that day, the four of us agreed that the absence of any real clinical data on this new procedure was real cause for concern, regardless of the initial results. Lyse was clearly uncomfortable with the lack of data and the fact that the treatment was still in its trial phase.

Dr. Anderson reviewed the side effects of the standard chemo regimen, and told us that the presence of small nodules left behind after surgery— she referred to it as "miliary disease"—was better than the presence of a tumor. She told Lyse that we needed to find a center, or hospital, that could provide the standard chemo regimen. She mentioned Hackensack University Hospital, and after that, Lyse could consider coming back to Sloan-Kettering for the trial therapy.

"You *can* choose to come here for chemotherapy," she added. "No matter who does it, the protocol will be the same. You may want to make your decision based on geographic location to make it easier for yourself, in terms of travel and physician appointments."

Before our meeting ended, Cathy asked the doctor about nutrition and diet.

"Well, if you feel like eating McDonald's, go for it," Dr. Anderson said lightly, looking at Lyse. "Go with what you feel like at this point."

What? What is she talking about?

I bristled at her off-the-cuff comment. Everyone knows that good nutrition is critical to good health. She may as well have said to Lyse, "Eat whatever the hell you want, because you already have the disease. It doesn't matter now."

On the way home, Lyse said, "I'd rather get my chemo close to home. If the protocol is the same all over, it makes sense to choose someplace that's close."

We all agreed, and Cathy suggested we contact Dr. Louis Attas, an oncologist at Holy Name Hospital in Teaneck, New Jersey. She went to him for her bleeding disorder, and she was crazy about him. Plus, the hospital was about fifteen minutes from our house. Lyse balked at Sloan's trial peritoneal therapy, but said she wouldn't make a final decision on that until she had completed her chemotherapy. She was interested in going to Holy Name for treatment.

Up until this point, Cathy had been researching top gynecologic physicians in the New York/New Jersey area. She had given the list to me. There were two out of Sloan-Kettering—Dr. Richard Barakat, who specialized in ovarian/uterine cancers, and Dr. William Hoskins, who specialized in ovarian/gynecologic cancers. Both physicians had been cited in New York Magazine's 2001 edition, under "Best Doctors in New York."

We arrived home around 4:00 p.m. Cathy and Joanne left for their house, and Lyse called Jeannine. My mom, Carolyn, had been with us since Saturday, October 5. She flew in from Sarasota and would stay until Sunday, the thirteenth, when Monique arrived. She was anxious to hear about our meeting with Dr. Anderson.

Mom had spent the day reading, doing our laundry, and taking care of Molly. They had taken a couple of walks around the neighborhood. Mom seemed comfortable in our home. That made me feel good.

Following dinner that night—Mom had prepared a satisfying meal of baked chicken, vegetables and a salad while we were out—I cleared the table and started the dishes. Mom stood on my right, and dried the dishes after I put them in the wooden drainer. After the washing was finished, I methodically wiped all the counters with a paper towel, scrubbed the sink with Ajax, and swabbed the back splash. I towel-dried the water spots around the sink.

My OCD had typically been a source of shame, and something I felt I had to hide and carry out in private. I always knew other people didn't clean and organize to the degree that I did. I didn't want people to know I was beholden to my compulsions to polish, neaten, and pigeonhole. I tried hard to scale back my actions when in front of others. However, doing so caused me even greater anxiety.

From the first, I felt safe enough with Lyse to fully disclose my infirmities—my blemishes. She didn't anger, didn't ridicule or pity me for it. To my amazement and complete relief, she let me do my thing. I vacuumed Fridays after work, and before we ate dinner. I ran the Dust Buster in the kitchen and hallway before we opened a bottle of wine for cocktail hour. Before we laid down for our Saturday afternoon nap, I vacuumed the crumbs Bridie had left behind. I swept the front porch steps before we took our bike ride. I straightened the couch cushions before we climbed the stairs to bed. She never angered, and never faulted me.

I could feel Mom's eyes on me. My arms stiffened in self-consciousness while I continued to rub the sink.

"Cher," she said.

I whirled around, feeling that maybe I was going to be scolded—our mother-daughter link snapping back thirty years in time.

I looked at her, expectantly.

"You need help, especially now." That was all she said.

I knew what she meant. Not the dishes, not Lyse, and not anything else. I needed help with my OCD. Much of the mother-daughter interchange transcended words. Eyes, facial expressions, and body language were imparted; words simply ferried the message, as a suitcase transports clothes. At least this was typical of our relationship.

We've never been close, nor distant. We've existed somewhere in the middle. Over time, the needle has moved much closer to close. My mother never received approval easily from her parents, and, I suppose, had carried on that tradition with her own children.

Love and approval go hand-in-hand when one is young and without understanding. Grasping that the two, for some, can be mutually exclusive, may be serendipitous, and healing.

When I finally deduced that Mom did love deeply, and that her love was not manifested through approval and coddling, I was resolved.

I wish I had figured it out sooner. The OCD personality repeats behavior until perfection is achieved. I tried to attain the approval I craved. It became a lifelong pursuit of perfection within our relationship.

"I think you need to talk with someone about your cleaning," she continued. "Your compulsion seems to be getting worse. You're going to get sick and fall apart if you don't get help. I'm worried about you."

My eyes teared up quickly as I supported myself against the counter, still clutching the damp paper towel.

"It's how I cope, Mom. It's how I deal with everything. It works for me," I replied, defending my defense, all the while accepting that she was right.

A small part of me was grateful I had been found out.

"A psychiatrist can give you the right medication so you can deal with Lyse's illness in a healthier way for yourself," she offered.

Her eyes pleaded with me. I felt what an addict at intervention must feel. I was a sitting duck. But I was also relieved.

"You're right," I replied. But, whatever drugs he's going to give me better not ruin my sleep or ability to do what I have to for Lyse," I grumbled.

"I'll talk to Phyllis," she offered.

Phyllis and Mom had met on the tennis courts in Sarasota and had been friends for a few years.

"Her cousin by marriage, Dr. Joelle Bunting, may be able to see you," she continued. "According to Phyllis, she's very good. I'm not sure she's taking new patients, but we'll see. I think this can really help you, Cher, and make things a little easier for you," she went on. "I don't like seeing you like this. Your own health has to come first."

"I know, I know. You're right," I replied, sighing with shoulders sagging. "I have a long road ahead of me and I know deep down that I can't continue at this pace."

She hugged me and turned to go upstairs to use the bathroom. Mom has had health issues of her own. Her ulcerative colitis nearly killed her in 1998. She now wears an iliostomy bag and is back on the tennis courts, leading a very active, and satisfying life.

While she went upstairs, I quickly ran for the Dust Buster and vacuumed the kitchen floor. I then dabbed a small amount of Murphy's Oil Soap on a white rag, and applied it to the top of the left side oak cabinet door under the sink. The garbage can sat behind this door. Lyse always opened the door by pulling the corner of the door instead of using the handle. From the constant rubbing, the top of the door dried out easily, so I had to moisturize it with wood soap all the time. Mom wasn't back yet, so I pulled out the garbage can from its slider caddy, and wiped off the crumbs that had accumulated on the floor of the holder. My heart pounded and my breaths came in gasps. I quickly put the can back in the holder, threw away the soiled paper towel, and closed the cabinet door, with the handle.

My sisters rallied around us also. They drove up from Princeton to see us about three-and-a-half weeks after Lyse had had her surgery. Lyse was still recovering but was able to move about the house again. Lisa, and Deb, younger than me by two and three years respectively, were ready and available for me as I came to accept the magnitude of the burden Lyse and I had just been handed.

The three of us went down the street to the River Edge Diner for lunch. I was barely hungry. I ordered something I could pick at that would be somewhat nutritious without being too nauseating—egg salad on a kaiser roll, and a Coke.

I had already lost a couple of pounds; my adrenaline was burning up calories faster than I could consume them.

My sisters and I were close, and always had been. During the tumultuous years we lived with Sidney—after he and Mom were married in 1973—we bonded even more tightly.

Deb became a nurse. At a young age, she married and had Dan, and then Katie. Lisa waited a few years to marry and start her family. When Lyse got sick, Benjamin was five years old. He and Lyse had made a solid connection. Ben even gave Lyse her own branch on his genealogy tree in elementary school.

Sisters as close as we were did not fail to mark the subtlest of changes in one another. A combination of eagle eyes and years of witnessing the good, bad and ugly in each other meant we were enlightened instantly, through a slight inflection in the voice, a faint pull of the mouth, or an awkward turn of the head.

The sisterly kinship, then, continually quickened and deepened. We didn't have to interpret communiqué. It cinched our ability to get down to the real business of sharing, conjecturing, and helping.

Lisa and Deb entered into my grief and fear that day. They helped me hold it up for a little while. Lisa was optimistic because she wanted me to be. Deb was cautiously optimistic because she knew better.

"Why *wouldn't* the chemo kill the cancer?" I asked Deb, as if its success were a given.

She didn't speak. Her unspoken reply was articulate, and quite translucent.

"It may not. This is a bad cancer."

Her years of nursing, working in the trenches, infirmities and sickliness, had betrayed her sisterly support.

The egg salad lurched in my stomach. I leaned back from my plate. For a moment, we all just sat there and said nothing.

Lisa did our grocery shopping several times. She would drive up from Princeton while Ben was in school, fulfill our list at Shop-Rite in Paramus, cart everything home to us, and unpack it.

She and Deb did our shopping the day we went to lunch, including the wine shopping.

They sent cards and e-mails to Lyse regularly. They sent cards to me. Words of encouragement, support and love always seemed to come at the times we needed them most.

CHAPTER SIX:
DOWN TO A SCIENCE

Wednesday, October 23, 2002

This morning we met with Dr. Lewis Attas, from Holy Name Hospital's Regional Cancer Center. Cathy and Joanne were with us. We showed up armed with notebooks, pens, and a hefty amount of questions. A short, stocky man in his late fifties, the doctor's demeanor was jovial, relaxed and easy going. We immediately felt at ease.

He was engaging, warm and energetic. He welcomed our questions and answered all of them in detail. He was thrilled to see that Lyse had a solid support system, and embraced our presence with her. He had a decent sense of humor, and was completely disarming. I think we all knew pretty quickly that we had found the right oncologist. We later agreed that we needed to look no further.

He spent a good deal of time reviewing Lyse's medical history. He touched on everything and missed nothing. He had read her records ahead of time and impressed us with his detailed knowledge of her surgical and test results.

He explained that when tumor cells are found in the fluid of the abdominal cavity, chemotherapy is necessary. Without dwelling on the diagnosis, he stated that Lyse's condition was considered "Stage 3C." In Stage 3 of the disease, the cancer has moved beyond the pelvis into the omentum. Stage 3C means that the tumors found in the abdomen are larger than 2 cm in size. There are four defined stages of the disease. In fact, according to cancerhelp. org, most cancers are categorized into four stages, and there may be further delineation within stages, depending on the type of cancer.

He expressed his frustration at the lack of available screening yet reassured us that "the biggest strides have been in surgery." He stated that peritoneal, not ovarian cancer, may have been the primary disease in Lyse's case, "which is maybe why it wasn't detected." Treatment is the same for both.

"Your surgery seemed good," he went on to say optimistically, while looking directly at Lyse.

I was pleased with his eye contact.

He outlined the main points of treatment. A total of six infusions would be given, spaced three weeks apart. Calendar elapsed time would be about four and one-half months, give or take a week or two for holidays and scheduling.

Lyse would be pre-medicated with steroids the night before, and given an antihistamine the morning of infusion. She might experience nausea and vomiting, mostly during day one. The steroids would help minimize sickness after treatment. She would lose her hair in about three weeks, but could expect full regrowth upon completion of the treatment.

His recommendations included working with the nutritionist at the cancer center, for healthy and agreeable meal ideas after treatment and in-between infusions. He suggested that she should purchase a wig, for comfort in public. Cathy later told us that Cedar Lane in town was full of wig shops. They catered to Orthodox Jewish women who required all manner of head coverings. She assured us that we'd be able to find a wig and some colorful and interesting scarves and hats.

Dr. Attas concluded by reviewing the follow-up procedures that we could expect after completing all rounds of treatment—a CT scan every four months and routine blood work to check cancer counts.

We asked him one of our most pressing questions: "Does intra-peritoneal therapy work?"

We discovered that "the trials are not suggesting a second look." A second look means examining the peritoneal cavity via laparoscope in conjunction with the IP therapy.

"I haven't seen data that supports IP therapy after chemotherapy," he replied, in a manner that made it clear he wouldn't use a protocol that hadn't been proven.

Wednesday, October 30, 2002

Today's the day. Chemo, round one. As instructed, Lyse took four Decadron (dexamethasone) tablets—small, white square pills—last night at dinner, and four more with breakfast this morning. This medication was used to relieve inflammation and allergic reactions. She had trouble sleeping last night.

Side effects as noted on the CVS Pharmacy Patient Prescription Information: May cause dizziness, nausea, indigestion, increased appetite, weight gain, weakness or sleep disturbances.

Other than a spotty night's sleep, she felt pretty good this morning. Her complexion was good, as was her spirit.

Our appointment was at 8:00 a.m. I had requested a day off so I could support her, and reassure her. Perhaps I could even distract her from this rather spooky procedure which involved a seven-hour dump of chemicals into her bloodstream. She was nervous about the whole process and even more uncomfortable about the side effects of the drugs.

To access the Regional Cancer Center, we used the same driveway the ambulances used for the emergency room. The center sat parallel to the emergency room, further down the driveway. We entered the revolving door—the set of regular doors was reserved for those in wheelchairs—and were greeted by the first floor receptionist. She told us to take the elevator to the second floor, where we would find the infusion center.

Holy Name Hospital has served northern Bergen County, New Jersey, for over eighty years. Its specialties include: dialysis treatment, cancer care, women's health services, radiology treatment, cardiovascular treatment and neurology services.

The hospital was founded by the Sisters of St. Joseph of Peace, in 1925, and is affiliated with the New York-Presbyterian Health System. My workplace, conveniently, was a seven-minute drive from the hospital.

The infusion center's receptionist, Marina, greeted us with a sparkly smile when we exited the elevator. The front desk was appointed with tasteful flower arrangements and a small dish of colorful hard candies. The waiting area was dressed in soothing greens, beiges, and muted blues. A small wrought iron fountain gurgled and splashed delicately. There were four comfortable armchairs in the corner and organized piles of magazines like *National*

Geographic and *Country Living* resting on small tables. The magazines were glossy and inviting; crisp corners implied the staff's attention to detail in all areas of patient comfort.

Eileen, the intake nurse, took Lyse's vital signs—blood pressure, pulse, and temperature. She also drew blood. Before an infusion was started, blood was checked for anemia (low red blood cell count) and neutropenia (low white blood cell count) that decreased the patient's ability to fight infection. If counts were not where they needed to be, chemotherapy was postponed. Lyse's blood work and vitals looked good. Eileen walked us down the hall, past Dr. Attas's office, to the infusion center. Lyse was wearing her black, tailored, dress pants from Lands End, the sage silk shirt I had given her for Christmas a year ago, and black loafer-style shoes. She really looked sharp. She told me she wanted to dress well for her treatments, saying that looking good translated into feeling good.

Cheryl was Lyse's nurse for the day. She greeted us warmly. Her years of patient care were evident from the way she engaged us solidly, and confidently. She had pleasant brown eyes and dark blonde hair cut in a bob. Her stocky build was perhaps a result of goodies from grateful families, or carbohydrate-rich cafeteria food. Pink scrub pants and a brightly flowered nurse's top complemented her good cheer and sparked our comfort.

She gave us a brief tour. In the main room, the nurse's station was surrounded by eight infusion chairs that were spaced apart at a comfortable distance. Each chair had a privacy curtain. None were drawn. Two rooms in the back were reserved for those patients requiring more intimate care during infusion, or who had become ill during treatment.

There was a small, sunny kitchen off to the side with a sink, table and well-stocked refrigerator. Snack packages of vanilla and chocolate pudding, milk, juice, ice cream, sherbet, yogurt, and cheeses were stacked neatly on the shelves.

Crackers, granola bars, napkins, paper plates and plastic cutlery could be found in the cabinets above the sink. Everything was organized, clean, and welcoming. The bathroom was on the other side of the room; the oversized layout accommodated patients and their IV poles.

Since this was Lyse's initial treatment, she would be seated directly across from the nurse's station, for close observation by the staff.

"Are you ready, Lyse?" Cheryl asked with an affectionate, reassuring smile.

"I'm as ready as I'm going to be," Lyse replied, smiling, and a little calmer now.

"Well," Cheryl continued, "we're going to get you comfortable in your chair, and then we can get started. We'll be by your side for the whole thing."

Lyse settled herself in the armchair—bright fabric and soft, ample seating beckoned—and Cheryl reviewed the procedure for the day.

"First," she said, "we're going to give you Benadryl, intravenously. That's for any possible allergic reactions. We'll also give you a small dose of Ativan to help you relax. Then we'll start the medicine. The first bag will take a few hours, and the second one takes about an hour. So, you'll know, once I put the second bag on, you're almost finished."

Cheryl's strong New York area accent was somehow comforting and disarming all at once. Because she was upfront yet casual and unassuming about the process, Lyse visibly relinquished some of her pent-up stress.

"You, OK, babe?" I asked gently after Cheryl left to gather the medication.

Lyse smiled at me and responded, "I'm doing pretty well, actually. I feel very comfortable with the people here. We'll just take it as it comes."

Lyse didn't rush things, or jump to conclusions, quickly. She was very measured in her thinking and responses. A male colleague had once told her that she "thought like a man." She possessed a favorable and unique blend of cerebral and emotional intelligence, and managed life challenges with a very impressive synthesis of the two.

She would go on to manage her illness in much the same way.

"I don't want you to worry, sweetie," I offered reassuringly. "I'll be with you all day, right by your side. Remember, we're doing this together."

Two other patients had joined us at this early hour. One woman, possibly in her late sixties, was wearing tastefully applied makeup, and was immaculately dressed in colorful prints and a deep rust-colored wig. Sparkly gold earrings, bracelets, and rings dangled from every limb. She smiled, cordially, at Lyse and me as she came in alone, then she promenaded confidently over to a chair at the end of our row.

Cheryl greeted her warmly, and told her that Laurie, the other nurse, would be over shortly to take care of her.

"She looks like she knows the ropes," Lyse commented.

"She seems very comfortable," I replied lightly.

I could tell that Lyse was really encouraged by the cosmopolitan attire and poised air of the woman.

Another lady sat across from us, with a young man who could have been her son. She appeared to be of Middle Eastern descent, with olive skin, black hair and almond eyes. She was dressed comfortably in a light blue sweatsuit and white sneakers. Rather quiet and withdrawn, she spoke to her son in terse snippets of dialogue.

73

Cheryl returned with the medication, and hung the bags on the hooks of the IV pole. She rolled up Lyse's right sleeve, sterilized the injection site, and searched for a vein.

"My veins are tough to find, and they're small," Lyse said. She didn't grimace, or wince.

Cheryl said, "Well, they're not going to get tricky on us. They're going to behave," she replied, smiling, as she punctured the vessel successfully.

A half hour later, the Benadryl and Ativan infusions were completed. Lyse was sleepy. Closing her eyes, she leaned her head back on the soft headrest. Cheryl switched out the empty bags for the plastic packs of Taxol and Carboplatin. She started the first drip. I scanned the literature we had been given.

"Taxol is an antineoplastic used to treat cancer," the fact sheet from Holy Name's pharmacy read. According to the American Heritage Dictionary, an antineoplastic acts by "inhibiting or preventing the growth or development of malignant cells."

The fact sheet stated: *"SIDE EFFECTS, that may go away during treatment, include flushing, nausea, vomiting, diarrhea, or mild muscle and joint pain. If they continue or are bothersome, check with your doctor. YOUR HAIR MAY FALL OUT while you are receiving this medication. It usually grows back after you stop treatment. CHECK WITH YOUR DOCTOR AS SOON AS POSSIBLE if you experience fever or chills, numbness or tingling of your hands or feet, fever, skin rash, difficulty breathing, or unusual or unexplained bruising or bleeding. If you notice other effects not listed above, please contact your doctor, nurse, or pharmacist."*

Lyse's primary, and most debilitating complaint—not listed above—was fatigue—a crippling fatigue which led to a coma-like sleep—a sleep that would suffocate her and leave her dormant for three days at a time.

I'd rouse her periodically and hold her arm while she shuffled to the bathroom. I'd wake her regularly and give her teaspoons of water and red nausea-control pills. I'd lay next to her on the bed to see that her chest was moving, and to make sure I heard any small sound of breathing. It seemed she was only one shallow breath away from certain death. It appeared she was in a sleep so bottomless that the only way out was down.

On the fourth day, she would stir. She was able to tolerate small sips of chicken broth which I gave to her from a mug. She sat on the living room couch and watched *Ellen*, and *Oprah*. She would say the nausea was receding and she'd smile. I'd feel relieved; she'd feel grateful. Her eyes would shine. We'd savor those early moments of awakening, and were jubilant. She was out of the woods for another two-and-a-half weeks.

By day five, Lyse would eat my homemade "special soup," as we called it—tiny diced carrots and celery with a little rice simmered in chicken broth—which gave her some strength. She'd enjoy the smell of the soup and would look forward to small mugs of it throughout the day.

We came to expect the post-infusion unfolding of events as they were. From the predictability came comfort.

By day six, it was as if Lyse had never undergone treatment of any kind. The flush would vanish from her face. She'd have strength and would want to move about, pay bills, talk on the phone, and putter in the kitchen.

We'd walk Molly around the neighborhood, and visit the local nursery to pick out decorations for the front garden. Cathy and Joanne would come over and we'd enjoy wine, cheese and soft conversation. Lyse would allow herself a couple sips of my red wine and then she'd switch to grape juice. We'd enjoy those routine moments in our life with renewed heartiness.

The first drip continued throughout the morning and into the afternoon. Lyse tolerated the medicine well, and had settled into the tedious and wearisome process.

Drip. Drip. Drip. The room had since quieted. The patients passed their time reading, dozing and gazing at TV talk shows that hummed like small motors from each chair. Every quarter hour, Cheryl and Laurie quietly strode from station to station. Their sneakers pattered across the floor as they checked on monitors and medicine levels. Infusion bags squished at their touch. They tended to their paperwork at the desk, and spoke to each other in hushed tones. The turn of glossy pages in a magazine, a spoon tapping against a Styrofoam sherbet cup, a wrapper crinkling as it was pulled off of a granola bar—the ordinary sounds were titillating, and took on a sponginess which melded into a bubbling stew of gentle sonance that hypnotized me, caressed my ears and made me sleepy.

At 2:30 p.m., Cheryl started the second drip. Lyse had been feeling pretty good all day. For lunch, she enjoyed a peanut butter sandwich and a carton of whole milk. After Cheryl changed the bag, Lyse asked me for a cup of apple juice. I was grateful she had not had a bad reaction to the drugs thus far and was experiencing an uneventful first treatment.

This day, with its sequence of steps and processes that we needed to execute carefully, reminded me of my first, and only, time rock climbing the Shawangunk Mountains of Ulster County, New York. Anxiety preceded each step that I took up the face of the rock. Locking into a firm toehold in a crescent-shaped notch sent a warm wave of relief burbling out from my spine to my limbs.

The relief was quickly replaced by anxiety about searching for the next toehold, as I crawled higher—the woman below looking more like an insect than my lover.

Dovetailing anxiety and release filled my being throughout Lyse's first day of treatment. Watching her receive and endure the therapy put me back on that rock in the Shawangunks. It was a cycle of worry and relief, each roused by the other. My limbs grew weary this day, also.

The second drip was short and Cheryl told us we would be finished by about 4:00 p.m. Dr. Attas stopped by mid-afternoon and greeted Lyse heartily. She was thrilled to see him and very pleased that he had made the effort to check on her.

He was all smiles and warmth—a teddy bear in a lab coat.

"When's Cheryl going to let you out of this medieval torture device?" he said, grinning, and gesturing to the IV pole.

"As soon as you give her the go ahead!" Lyse replied, smiling back.

The doctor and Lyse had connected. He had a son in eighth grade. Lyse taught seventh grade. He talked about the science program at his son's school. She described highlights of the science curriculum at her school. They compared notes and shared an easy banter. She appreciated his corny humor and bad puns. So did I.

He turned to leave and reminded Lyse about her next appointment with him for blood work results.

"And don't forget to come in tomorrow for your Neulasta shot," he continued. "No sleeping in," he said, grinning. "I know how you teachers get when you're off work."

His wiry, curly hair looked unkempt and sprung out in all directions from his receding hairline.

"Will do," she replied, smiling broadly.

The Neulasta injection boosted white blood cell counts to help the body fight infection that might otherwise easily take hold in a being weakened by chemotherapy drugs.

Lyse turned to look at me and said, "Well, we're almost there. It wasn't as bad as I thought. The nurses make all the difference. Cheryl was wonderful."

"You've done so well today, baby," I replied. "I'm so proud of you. We're so lucky to have such an amazing medical team."

She continued, "When I close my eyes, I picture the chemo drugs as white light going into my veins—white light that will kill the cancer and flush it out of me."

I smiled and nodded.

"That's really great, babe. Focusing on the white light is healing and therapeutic. I'm so glad you're doing that. I am, too. When I see your abdomen in my mind's eye, I picture white light just bathing that whole area and smothering the cancer cells. It's very real and powerful."

Two hours later, with the "all clear" from Cheryl, we were on our way home. We were both energized, and even buzzed a little—Lyse, from the steroids and success of the day, and me, from the intensity of Lyse undergoing treatment and the responsibility of keeping her comfortable and protected so she could heal.

At 4:45 p.m., we arrived home. There was a message from Jeannine, one from Cathy and Joanne, and one from Camille. Lyse called Jeannine right away and filled her in on the details of the day—the medication and how it was administered, how wonderful and caring the staff was, and how clean and comfortable we found the treatment area. Jeannine was jittery and overwrought. I could feel her strung-out energy through the phone line. It angered me. Lyse reassured her that all was going well and she shouldn't worry.

I wanted to grab the phone and blurt out, "Get a grip! There's no good use for your jumpiness right now. Get a hold of yourself! Calm down! It's stressful for Lyse to have to manage your anxiety as well!"

In retrospect, I think calming Jeannine may have helped Lyse quiet herself. Energy focused on another's angst means less time to dwell on one's own.

When I returned home from work the next day, Lyse started to feel sick. When I spoke with her from the office, her voice sounded raspy and thin. I knew something was coming.

She was sitting on the couch, looking pale and sapped. I could see the effects of yesterday's chemo setting in, reaching to consume her like spilled ink on a bright sheet of parchment paper. She couldn't think of food. Dinner was out of the question. She wanted to fall into bed and sleep. I walked with her upstairs, pulled down the bed while she undressed, and then tucked her in. The time was 6:00 p.m.

She vomited twice that night, and then slept until Sunday. I roused her to give her sips of water, red nausea pills—Compazine—and to help her to the bathroom.

She was coherent by Sunday morning. I sat on the edge of the bed and smiled at her, kissed her hand, and kissed her lips and forehead. I hugged her and told her I loved her.

"Wow," she mumbled, "I guess I've been sleeping, huh?"

"Yes, babe, you've been sleeping soundly. It's Sunday morning."

"No, it can't be," she replied with alarm, her eyes widening.

"Baby, it's OK. You started getting sleepy Thursday night and your body needed to rest. It's okay. All that matters is that you're feeling better now," I offered gently, while smiling.

As we talked quietly, I was overcome with a wretched feeling of sadness, a sorrow for what my partner must endure. I was filled with a cavernous hollow carved by the sharpness of my grief.

When I knew I'd spend the rest of my life with her, I made a promise to Lyse's spirit guide, a Native American Indian whose presence she felt in times of trouble. He had saved her life when she was an infant in 1941. Her family lived next to an Indian reservation in the Canadian countryside. When her mother developed complications during Lyse's birth, her father sent for the city doctor.

The doctor told Lyse's father that at such a fragile size Lyse likely wouldn't make it, and that he had better put his energies into saving his wife. Besides, he had pointed out, they already had five other children. The doctor later bundled Lyse's spindly body into the rags and towels being discarded. Georgette uncovered Lyse's body from outside, brought her back in, and had her younger brother, Guilles, run for the medicine man next door on the reservation.

The shaman tended to Lyse and built her a makeshift incubator in the oven. Her father fed her with an eyedropper and she stayed warm in her oven basket for a few weeks. She grew, and then grew stronger. Several visits later, once he knew she was stable, the medicine man stopped coming. The family never saw him again. Lyse sensed him at her side, then, and in the years that followed.

I felt him, too. By June 1996, two months after our first date, I knew I would spend the rest of my life with Lyse. In the darkness of my living room late one night, I felt the presence of the medicine man. In my mind's eye, I saw his ceremonial robes, jewelry and headdress. I dropped to my knees and told him that I loved Lyse, and would take care of her for the rest of her life. I sensed he needed to know that before he could continue on his spiritual path. I reassured him that with me she would be safe, would be loved, and would be protected. After that, I never felt his presence again.

"Babe, if I could switch with you, I would. I should be the one in the bed so I can spare you from all of this. I want to take on this battle for you," I said deliberately, solemnly, and with tears climbing up my rib cage from the depths of my sorrow, stinging my torso and throat, and working their way to my eyeballs.

Love is given, and then love is taken away. We play witness to both, nothing more. We try hard to forget about the end part, hoping that the day never comes, thinking that the time is so far off, surely something will save us from that fate. It's the unthinkable destiny of losing the one person who makes our life worth living passionately, the way it should be lived.

I had hoped we'd go together. I told Lyse I didn't want to go without her, nor did I want to stay behind after she left. I'd never felt that way before. It froze me to think about not being with her—like the way I felt when my parents pulled away after dropping me at summer camp. Panic and fear smothered me in desperation. The grief was so deep it obliterated my sense of self.

November 13, 2002

Lyse's hair began to fall out today. She noted this in her Yorkie calendar—"hair loss"—next to "good day" since she had indeed felt good that day, except for the hair loss. It had been exactly two weeks to the day from her first infusion. Dr. Attas had said it would all fall out within three weeks. It didn't come out at once. It came out in clumps, clusters of ten to twenty soft, silver strands at a time. They blanketed the hardwood floors, the marble tile of the master bath, and her pillow. It seemed there was more hair on the floor than matched the bald patches on her head.

It didn't make sense. The only thing I could figure was that there was more hair on the human head than we estimated. From the looks of it, there would be tons more hair under our feet before all was said and done. I couldn't get my arms around this one. I just had to wait, then vacuum, wait, and then vacuum again. I couldn't anticipate when the strands would fall. I was beholden to the schedule of those little follicles. I wanted it to be over. One big vacuum, and done.

No, it was a little bit here, and a little bit there. Randomly, day or night, they fell. I was on constant lookout for any fresh casualties.

I was anxious for Lyse; it was driving her crazy, also. She was afraid, uncomfortable, and unsettled. I wanted to make it better for her. For her sake, I just wanted it over. She had her hair trimmed by MaryAnn, our hairdresser in Teaneck, the day after it started. It helped a little, but was raggedy by the next day.

Cathy and Joanne came over on Sunday, the seventeenth. They brought Toby, their second oldest Yorkie, with them. He and Molly romped for a while, and then they fell asleep at our feet. We had wine and cheese, and talked, as we lounged on the floor in front of the crackling fireplace. Lyse talked a little about her hair loss. She was sad about it, and clearly shaken.

Cathy looked at Lyse and blurted out, "Why don't we just shave it all off and be done with it? You won't have to agonize about it for another two weeks!"

"What a great idea!" I replied, looking at Lyse. "Sweetie, you'll get it over with quickly, and we'll be here right by your side. You'll never have this much fun getting a haircut!"

"Well, I don't know," Lyse said softly. "Maybe it's a good idea, but I don't know if I'm ready." She sighed deeply, a forlorn look clouding her face. "Plus, who will shave me?"

"Joanne will, of course!" Cathy jumped in. "She's the shaving queen, the razor expert! She shaves dogs all the time at work before giving them shots," Cathy continued. "She'll just pretend you're a client!"

We all burst out laughing.

"Okay, let's do it," Lyse said, brightening. "You're right. It's better to get it over with now and have a little fun while we're at it." She smiled.

"This shaving party is officially underway!" Cathy belted out, as she walked over to the stereo and cranked up the volume.

I refilled the wine glasses and topped off Lyse's glass with more grape juice. The dogs ran around the living room, chasing each other and panting with excitement at the festiveness.

I set up a chair in the middle of the kitchen and spread the morning newspaper on the floor, while Cathy draped Lyse in two towels from the downstairs linen closet. Joanne readied the razor which she had fetched from her vet bag in the car.

Lyse sat quietly. We all stood around her, circling her like prairie wagons harboring an injured member of the clan. Joanne slowly worked the razor up Lyse's neck, to the back of her ears, and then around the orb of her head.

Cathy and I kissed each new bald spot, hugging her head to our torsos. Lyse said the razor tickled.

Thirty minutes later, Lyse's head shone brightly under the kitchen light. We all clapped and cheered, showering her with kisses.

"You've got a hell of a perfect head, girlfriend," Cathy remarked while grinning. "It's perfectly round and just adorable! We should all be so lucky."

"Whoo, hoo baby!" I hooted. "Aren't you the cutest thing? I hope you're going my way!" I said, smooching her loudly on the lips.

"Thank you," Lyse said quietly, smiling. "Nice to know my head is really the sexiest part of me!"

She walked into the powder room with Cathy and I in tow, and looked in the mirror. I watched as she looked at herself.

"Oh, wow," she murmured, sliding her fingers across her newly shorn globe. "It's not too bad, really. I guess I can live with this."

I saw her eyes fill up. A couple of tears dribbled onto her cheeks from underneath her glasses. Her disease was robbing her of one thing at a time. This loss seemed to hit her the hardest.

❧

I wondered how it would be if *I* had had to endure such a loss. Lyse's connection to her hair, as to most things in her life, were healthy and normal. My association with my hair was a fiery amalgamation of my anxieties, fears and need to control.

The more Sidney tamped us down with house rules and canons during those years in Ventnor, the more my hair served as a whipping boy—a sacrificial lamb of sorts—for my anger about his oppressive rule. The panic and dread that went hand-in-hand with not angering him, and obeying all the rules, showcased itself in the frenzied, almost violent, way I handled my mane.

Managing my hair on a daily basis became a full-time obsession. From the moment I woke up until I crawled into bed at night, weighed down mercilessly with bobby pins, nothing was as important as getting my hair molded into the perfect shape.

I had inherited my father's persnickety hair. His locks were curly also, but the corkscrews looked good on him, framing his boyish smile and blue eyes well. As he grew older, though, the dark curl turned to gray frizz, and the top of his head was transformed from fertile terrain to a sparsely populated dustbowl—which even his comb-over, a right-to-left doohickey thing—couldn't salvage.

Riding with the window down had been a shameful experience for the rest of the family as "the piece" quickly came undone and stood straight out the window—a withered claw grasping desperately at passing cars and neighbors.

Years later, living with our new stepfather, my sisters and I were forbidden to use the hair dryer in the mornings before school.

"Only Margate snobs use those," Sidney had stated.

Margate was the town next to ours. Lots of rich Jewish kids, with doctor or attorney parents, lived there.

No hair dryer, and curly but frizzy-when-humid hair was a losing proposition, especially for a seventeen-year-old girl. In the pre-dawn hour, I had to make do with crude, but quiet tools like combs, ugly barrettes and curling irons that I used to angrily flatten the offending waves, scalding my scalp in the process.

Most mornings, I was forced to wash my hair, as sleeping on my short tresses ruined what had been the perfect coif the day before. The early morning hair-wash ritual had to be done quickly, quietly, and stealthily. Waking Sidney at that hour would have been an unthinkable transgression. My OCD, my meticulous care in keeping quiet and creeping through the grooming process, actually guaranteed my success. My OCD enabled me to carry out and survive the tortuous scene. It all began at 5:00 a.m., with the soft *brrrrr* of my alarm.

First, from bed to floor. Like a skilled gymnast, I swung my legs out of bed, and noiselessly landed on the portion of non-creaky flooring, two and a half steps from the door, and a half step to the left. Done. No stirring from Mom and Sidney's bedroom directly below. I sucked in a quick breath and congratulated myself.

I began the journey to the bathroom. I was grateful for the wind picking up outside and could feel my taut hamstrings loosening slightly.

"One, two, three, four steps, I'm in," I murmured, my heart ramming my breastbone.

The cold linoleum stung my bare feet and caused my eyes to bug. I closed the door and turned on the light switch. I breathed several more times. My breaths were shallow and quick. All clear from below. I heard Sidney's snoring.

"That's good," I whispered with relief.

I turned on the hot faucet—a centimeter's turn at first so as not to raise a stream of noisy air up the pipes and awaken the house! Slowly. Slowly.

I turned the hot water faucet only three-quarters of the way. I knew that opening it any further would spill a larger stream that would swish loudly down the drain. Three-quarters or less meant there would be no sound. Perfect. I let it run until the water was warm.

"Hurry, you f* * * * * g old house pipes!"

I took several more shallow, quick breaths. Next, I padded back to the hall to check for any stirring below. Everything was quiet. I filled up the plastic sixty-four ounce pitcher, while tilting it twenty-three degrees to counteract the swish. I think I heard *him*.

"Oh, my god," my voice screamed inside my head. "Stop the water, stop now, *stop now*."

Standing frozen over the faucet, I had trouble listening due to the ringing in my ears and the pounding between my breasts.

"Damn it," I whispered angrily.

A toilet flushed and feet plodded back to bed.

"He's just going to the bathroom! Yeah!" I roared excitedly in my mind.

With the plastic container full of water, I crept over to the metal shower stall. Pulling the curtain aside, I bent down, with my knees on the rug, and poured the warm water over my rumpled head. It felt so good. The water tickled and its warmth sent goose bumps down my taut, cold back. My concentration lost, I poured the water too quickly. It crackled in the drain.

"Crap, crap, crap!" I scolded myself in an angry whisper. "Go more slowly." I placed the pitcher down on the rug. I lathered my achy head and then padded back to the sink, and filled the pitcher again. After rinsing all of the suds, I grabbed the towel, released my breath, and wrapped the terry around my sopping head.

"Done, done, done!" I whispered excitedly to myself.

I enjoyed a moment of peace, and then turned around too quickly.

My right elbow whacked the shower wall. The cheap metal siding of the shower banged like a cymbal in a Fourth of July parade. Fear careened wildly through my pulsing, throbbing veins, like a wrecking ball, smashing the relief I felt just seconds ago. Stirring came from the bedroom below. The bed creaked as Sidney arose.

"Oh my god, I'm done for. It's over. I'm finished," I whispered in a choked voice as my knees weakened and my stomach soured.

"Who's up there?" Sidney barked. "Who's up there?"

It was 5:19 a.m.

"I had to get up early to wash my hair," I whimpered from the top of the landing. "I tried to be very quiet." Tiny hairs bristled on my still damp neck.

My hair had started to dry in the towel and I'd already lost my chance to mold it under the bobby pins. I felt my pounding heart in my stomach.

"People in this house are sleeping at this hour!" his booming voice echoed side-to-side up the stairs, and reached out toward me like a scythe slicing the air.

"Where is your consideration?" he continued loudly. "Next time, think of the other people in this house and not just yourself!"

"Okay," I choked. My stomach lurched.

In a huff, Sidney retreated to his bedroom and I quickly undid my head-towel. If I hurried and got my hair tamped down under the bobby pins, it still might turn out okay for school. My heart raced as small beads of perspiration dotted my forehead.

Lyse told me all the time that she thought I was beautiful. The first time she said it, I was so rattled, and so unbelieving, I just mumbled, "No, I'm not." No partner had ever told me that before. I know now that those partners were unable to step outside of their own insecurities and their own issues enough to offer such pure and unconditional words of love.

That night, Lyse took my head in her hands, and said, "Cheryl, you are so beautiful. Don't let anyone ever tell you otherwise. You are beautiful inside and out. You may not have ever heard it from the people who should have told you so, but know that it is true."

It took me at least two years to really accept the compliment she gave me over and over again. Then, one day, it happened. I replied to her offering without thinking,

"Thank you, babe."

I didn't flinch. I didn't wince. I smiled. So did she.

We became old hands at the Carbo-Taxol curriculum. Lyse prepped with the steroids the night before, endured the eight hour infusion, slept for three days afterward, and took the red nausea pills I gave her. When she popped out of her sleep coma, she ate my "special soup," and went about paying her bills, reading, and catching up with friends and family. Outside of some on-again off-again diarrhea and a fickle appetite, Lyse was, for the most part, able to resume a fairly normal life.

My company, OSG Billing Services, was very good to me. My boss, Ed, director of technical services, and our human resources manager, Mike, permitted me to use a block of ninety non-consecutive family medical leave days, unpaid, at my discretion, whenever Lyse needed me.

That year, Lyse and I spent Christmas like we did every other year, except for the tree. We bought a small, pre-decorated artificial fir instead of hauling home the usual five-foot balsam from the local nursery. We put out the crèche— made from African olive wood—I had given Lyse three years before. It sat on the wooden coffee table.

Lyse had remarked that, "it looks like the holy family is springing right up out of the coffee table."

She loved the simplicity of that crèche—eight pieces in all. Baby Jesus in a tiny cradle, the kings, the animals, and Mary and Joseph. The suppleness of the smooth and rounded wood transformed the little sculptures into living, breathing creatures emanating an ethereal presence right there in our living room.

Lyse sent the oncology nurses, Nice, the P.A., and the front desk staff a holiday gift from Harry and David. Five decorative tins, in the shape of a snowman, were crammed with goodies such as chocolate covered cherries, gourmet pretzels and nuts, shortbread cookies and fruit-filled candies. I remember how much fun Lyse had picking out the perfect gift for her medical team; those who championed her fight; those who were intimate with the consequences of that fight. Neither the treatments, nor their side effects, ever cleaved our holidays. We were grateful.

So, life went on like this, quite predictably, until Lyse finally completed the last chemo infusion on Wednesday, February 12, 2003. She had had six infusions, in four months. We were optimistic about the long-term results as Lyse's cancer counts, over the course of treatment, had dropped dramatically. From counts in the 900s prior to cancer surgery, the numbers were at ten upon Lyse's completion of therapy. According to Dr. Attas, a count less than thirty-five meant there was no presence of cancer.

We rejoiced. We thanked god. We hugged and kissed each other and Molly. We were triumphant. We were cautiously optimistic and held ourselves in check. We had just crawled our way through a dank, serpent-like tunnel into the sunlight. We found ourselves squinting.

Wednesday, February 26, 2003

"Your choices are to watch and wait, or begin treatment of another drug right away," Dr. Attas explained.

"What do you suggest we do?" Lyse asked.

"In a case like yours, where we've seen such excellent blood results from treatment," Dr. Attas replied, "I typically recommend the watch and wait option. We will keep very close tabs on you during the watch and wait period. CA 125 tests and CT scans will be done on a regular basis, so, anything that does come up will be noticed and addressed right away."

"Hmmm," Lyse replied. She was flip-flopping the pros and cons as he spoke.

She and I looked at each other. Dr. Attas looked at us, one at a time, and an encouraging smile spread over his round face.

"What do you think, babe?" I asked her. "It's really our call now."

"I think I'd like to try the watch and wait and see how it goes," she replied matter-of-factly.

She was spent. She had had enough of the pills, the chemicals, the needles, the nausea, and the runs. I knew she needed the break. She wouldn't have agreed if she thought not continuing the chemo would harm her.

"I think it's a good idea, sweetie," I concurred. "You're going to be checked routinely, so if something does come up, we can jump on it right away."

She was jubilant. I was ecstatic. Jeannine was crestfallen. Later that day, Lyse had called her and told her the good news about the blood work. Then she told her the rest of the good news—no more chemo!

"No, Leeese, no," Jeannine had pleaded into the phone. "You can't stop the infusions now. This type of cancer is mean. It's aggressive, and may just come back if you don't continue with the medicine," she bemoaned.

Lyse explained that she would be tested regularly, and if something happened, they would catch it early. Jeannine tried repeatedly to get Lyse to change her mind that day, and all through the next two weeks. Lyse stuck to her decision.

❧

The Xanax knocked me out at night. I was at least guaranteed a reprieve of eight hours, and a chance to forget what was happening. The day we knew Lyse would have to undergo surgery, I called Dr. Zucker. I told him my partner likely had cancer, and that I needed something to help me manage the situation and the anxiety it produced. I knew I could survive if I just got my sleep.

I had been enjoying nights of fathomless, dreamless sleep since September, when the cancer trouble had started brewing. Dr. Zucker had agreed to write the prescription, with the understanding that the medication would help me manage the period of crisis.

According to the web site, webmd.com, Xanax is part of a class of drugs called benzodiazepines. These drugs affect the brain and central nervous system and have a calming effect. Tablets are available in doses of 0.25 mg, .50

mg, 1 mg, and 2 mg. The drug has the potential to cause addiction and should not be discontinued suddenly. Dr. Zucker gave me a thirty-day refillable supply of 0.25 mg tablets with instructions to take one tablet as needed, and not to exceed four tablets in a twenty-four-hour period.

Psyweb.com recommends a dose of 0.25 mg – .50 mg three times daily for treatment of anxiety and nervous tension. Total amounts within a twenty-four-hour period should not exceed 4 mg.

Although the Xanax helped me to sleep and curbed some of my anxiety, it didn't do a thing for my obsessive-compulsive reflexes.

As promised, Mom had placed a call to her friend, Phyllis, who contacted Dr. Joelle Bunting. I had begun seeing Dr. Bunting in October 2002. By March 2003, after some trial and error, we found the cure. During my first visit with Dr. Bunting, I had explained how I was coping with Lyse's illness. I told her all about the cleaning, the worrying, and how I was beholden to thoughts that whizzed round my brain and wouldn't stop.

I disclosed the scrubbing and cleaning I did in private. I described the constant fretting and told her it was just much worse now because Lyse was sick. She asked me many questions related to family history, and pertinent behavioral symptoms which I had encountered throughout my life.

"I'd like to give you something to help alleviate the OCD symptoms, and not just the anxiety," she offered gently.

"OCD?" I asked.

"Yes, what you are describing is obsessive-compulsive disorder," she replied. "It's no surprise that it has flared up even more so at this time, with Lyse being sick."

A tall and big-boned woman of Norwegian descent, she dwarfed her little writing desk behind which she sat during our sessions. Her blonde bob hung neatly at the bottom of her ears. Fair skin and freckles gave her sixty-something visage a youthful girl appearance that obvious wrinkles didn't even betray. She moved about gently and agilely, much to my surprise considering her girth. When she smiled, her brightly painted red lips revealed perfectly shaped sparkly teeth, the shine from which reflected in her ice-blue eyes.

I figured she wore plus-sized clothes, but didn't realize she maintained plus-sized office furniture as well, until I sat in the turquoise leather wing back chair. My smallish behind and short legs were gobbled up by the cavernous chair. In fact, my legs didn't even reach the beige carpeted floor, unless I scooted myself up to balance on the edge of the chair. I felt foolish and ridiculous—I shrank as I sat in the portly chair. All the other chairs were of the same corpulence. In the office of the ample, I was deflating right before my very eyes. I know how Lily Tomlin felt in that big chair on Rowan and Martin's Laugh-In.

"Let's try Anafranil," Dr. Bunting suggested.

"I've had allergic reactions to certain antibiotics and I'm nervous about trying new drugs," I said without hesitation.

"We're going to start you on a low dose, and then work our way up. It will be fine," she said reassuringly.

Anafranil is the brand name of clomipramine. According to mentalhealth. com: "...Clomipramine is a tricyclic agent with both antidepressant and anti-obsessional properties. Like other tricyclics, clomipramine inhibits norepinephrine and serotonin uptake into central nerve terminals, possibly by blocking the membrane-pump of neurons, thereby increasing the concentration of transmitter monoamines at receptor sites. Clomipramine is presumed to influence depression and obsessive and compulsive behavior through its effects on serotonergic neurotransmission. The actual neurochemical mechanism is unknown, but clomipramine's capacity to inhibit serotonin reuptake is thought to be important. Clomipramine appears to have a mild sedative effect which may be helpful in alleviating the anxiety component often accompanying depression."

In layman's terms, the drug would help curb my obsessive thoughts and compulsive behaviors.

After dinner that night, I took the first dose, and waited. I made it until 9:00 p.m. and then I started feeling a little weird. I told Lyse I was heading to bed. On my way upstairs, I had the sensation that I was moving about in someone else's body. I felt disconnected from myself, as if I were not me anymore. I climbed into bed, heart pounding, and tried to sleep. I couldn't drift off. My stomach started to lurch and I noticed rushes of adrenaline zipping up and down my limbs, sort of like a burning electrical current. The rushes lasted about thirty seconds and would then resume after twenty minutes or so. Lyse joined me in bed.

"Babe, I'm really scared," I choked out, looking over at her. I described the bizarre feelings.

"Your pupils look dilated," she stated, leaning closer to look at them.

"Oh, my god," I replied, my voice beginning to rise in panic.

I jumped out of bed and ran around the corner into the master bath to look at my eyes.

"Babe, you're right!" I exclaimed hysterically. "What's going on with this f* * * * *g medication?" I screeched as my oversized black pupils stared back at me in the mirror—like something from a horror film. I stood in the bathroom feeling as if I were floating out of my body. It was now 11:00 p.m. I tingled, then the rushes came, and then I vomited.

"Babe, I think I may just have to go to the emergency room. I feel so weird," I moaned. "I guess this is what a bad LSD trip must feel like. Thank you, Dr. Bunting, for trying to kill me."

"Come back to bed, sweetie," Lyse prodded. "You probably just need to sleep off the medicine. You can call Dr. Bunting in the morning and tell her you had a bad reaction."

I spent the rest of the night running to the bathroom with diarrhea and dry heaves. While in bed, I turned the nightlight on and off, every few minutes, to check the size of my pupils in my pocket mirror, to see if they were reducing at all. Obsession and panic begets the same. I endured the adrenaline rushes until the early morning hours, when they finally ceased. I had timed the rushes and knew how often they came, and how long they lasted. Not until early that afternoon did I finally come out of that terrifying trip. I was nauseous until the following day.

Thankfully, Lyse was on one of her good two weeks while I was tripping. There was only one toilet close to the bed. I reluctantly agreed to try another medication and had similar results. After that, I told Dr. Bunting no more psychedelic drugs.

She was not discouraged and told me we'd find the right thing. I stayed on the Xanax, bumping up my nightly dose to 3 mg, and then almost 4 mg. The old doses weren't strong enough anymore. She told me my dosage was higher than usual but knew it was short-term.

In February, Dr. Bunting encouraged me to try Lexapro.

"We're going to start you off with a grain, and then you'll stay on that for a couple of days. If it agrees with you, you can take a larger grain, and continue this process until you've inched your way up to 15 mg of Lexapro daily." It worked.

Within two weeks, I was up to 10 mg daily and experienced a profound decrease in the driving force behind my compulsive need to clean. I felt "suspended in time" as Dr. Bunting called it. I was able to be present in the moment, and was not tormented by whirling thoughts or worries. I felt as if a stack of bricks had just toppled from my shoulders.

"Is this how everyone feels?" I asked Lyse as we leisured over a tomato and basil pizza at Pizzeria Uno down the street from our house.

I felt liberated, free from the torment of my own thoughts, the dictate of having to scrub, polish and organize the house over and over again. Although the *need* to do these things didn't disappear, the *drive,* and the frenzy behind the need, subsided.

I often forgot about what I was supposed to be fretting about, and so, when I started worrying, the thought just vaporized and was gone. It was lost in a fuzzy blur of nothingness that stopped commanding my attention. I felt relief like I had never known. The worries that used to paralyze me, now tickled me for a few seconds, and then floated off as if they had never come at all.

It was hard to believe that countless years of tortuous worrying and obsessive cleaning could be quietly calmed within the span of two weeks. I considered it miraculous.

"We have it all," Lyse and I said, over and over again, during our eight years together.

We enjoyed life, in spite of its hardships and challenges. We traveled a lot in the beginning of our relationship. We took weekend trips to quaint towns like New Hope, Pennsylvania and Cape May, New Jersey. Our romantic getaways began on Friday evenings. We packed the car and then picked up sandwiches before getting on the highway. We talked and laughed during the drive. We gobbled our picnic dinner—turkey subs with lettuce, mayo, and provolone, chips, iced tea, and chocolate chip cookies—and drove to our destination under a hazy cloud of new love and giddiness.

As time went on, we traded our weekend trips for quiet weekends at home with Molly. We grilled fish or chicken and enjoyed brandy on our deck, under the stars. We spent hours at the park, and many more napping in the sunny alcove of the second floor spare bedroom on Saturday afternoons. We languished on Sundays in winter, lazing in front of the crackling fireplace, scouring the New York Times, and sipping deep goblets of Merlot.

Whether on the beach in Cape May, our deck in River Edge, or on the porch overlooking the Delaware River in Lumberville, Pennsylvania, our sentiments were the same.

"We have it all," we'd remark. Not boastfully, nor flippantly. Just gratefully. "We have our friends, family, each other, Molly, our home, our health, and our jobs."

We put aside the things that were worrying us at the time, and focused on all of the good in our lives. We knew we were blessed and we never hesitated to acknowledge it.

As I continued my life alone, years later, I was comforted by this, and comforted by the way in which we treasured and appreciated what we had been blessed with. It gave me sustenance to know we never wasted the time we had. The bounties we were given never went unrecognized.

I felt the type of strange deliverance akin to what a farmer must feel bundled with his family in the well-stocked cellar after a tornado wrecks his land and the life he's built.

Chapter Seven:
Keep On Keepin' On

Tuesday, July 1, 2003

"DOXIL?" Lyse repeated to Dr. Attas.

"Yes, it's called DOXIL," he replied, his brows knitted. "Based on the results of your recent blood tests, and CT scan, this therapy will be our next course of action."

DOXIL, as described on the doxil.com web site, is "indicated for the treatment of patients with ovarian cancer whose disease has progressed or recurred after platinum-based chemotherapy."

Dr. Attas had discovered, over the course of recent blood tests, that Lyse's cancer markers were beginning to soar. The web site continued to state, "A rise in CA-125 levels may seem troubling. However, CA-125 is only one of the many indicators of how you may be doing. A single CA-125 test is never definitive. For this reason, serial testing of CA-125 is very useful during therapy."

Dr. Attas had been closely monitoring Lyse's markers throughout March, April, May, and June. The numbers on the most recent tests were consistent, and irrefutable.

Lyse took it in stride. She didn't freak out, come unglued, cry, or sink into a hissy fit.

She simply said, "It is what it is."

She said we would take the necessary next steps as Dr. Attas instructed us.

Jeannine wasn't as judicious. Upon hearing the news from Lyse, she fretted, and bemoaned the fact that Lyse had not continued chemotherapy. Lyse told her she had made the best decision she could have at the time, and that we would deal with what was in front of us right now. When it came right down to it, I found her pragmatic and empirical approach to the hot potatoes of life rather refreshing.

What is DOXIL?

DOXIL is:

- *A chemotherapy drug used to treat or control cancer cells*
- *A different form of doxorubicin, a drug used to treat cancer*

How is DOXIL Different?

DOXIL is a reformulated version of doxorubicin. DOXIL takes the active agent doxorubicin and places it into a fat bubble called a liposome and another layer of hair-like strands made from methoxypolyethylene glycol—a type of rubber. This coating allows DOXIL to evade detection and destruction by the immune system which increases the time the drug is in the body. The majority of the drug stays inside the liposome while in the blood (at least 90%). Therefore, DOXIL has more time to reach the tumor tissue, where the medication slowly leaks out. However, DOXIL may also leak out and affect normal tissue.

www.doxil.com

July 3, 2003

Treatment with DOXIL may lead to cardiac toxicity and congestive heart failure, so patients are typically given a heart scan prior to beginning treatment. Lyse underwent a heart scan today and was given the thumbs up by Dr. Attas. Her first infusion was scheduled for Wednesday, July 9.

Generally, the drug was administered intravenously, once every four weeks, for a total of four cycles. Each infusion lasted about one hour. Lyse tolerated the new drug well.

So did the cancer.

September 17, 2003

Lyse's September 15 CT scan revealed that the three treatments of DOXIL she had received over the course of twelve weeks had done absolutely nothing to control the tumors. Her markers had not decreased; they were, in fact, on the rise.

Dr. Attas was visibly distraught with the assault of the malignant cells he was observing in Lyse's body. At our September 17 meeting with him, he explained that since DOXIL was not quelling the vicious and aggressive tumors, he advised that Lyse undergo treatment with a newer drug called GEMZAR, that would be given in combination with Cisplatin.

GEMZAR is a chemotherapy drug used to treat certain kinds of cancer. GEMZAR works by stopping the process that cells use to divide and repair themselves, leading to cell death.

www.Gemzar.com

Cisplatin (sis-PLA-tin) belongs to the group of medicines known as alkylating agents. It is used to treat cancer of the bladder, ovaries, and testicles. It may also be used to treat other kinds of cancer, as determined by your doctor.

Cisplatin interferes with the growth of cancer cells, which are eventually destroyed. Since the growth of normal body cells may also be affected by cisplatin, other effects will also occur. Some of these may be serious and must be reported to your doctor. Other effects may not be serious but may cause concern. Some effects may not occur for months or years after the medicine is used.

www.Mayoclinic.com

Clinical Oncologists for Individualized Treatment of cancer patients have found out years ago that the combination of gemcitabine + platinum (either cisplatin, carboplatin or oxaliplatin) was the most important drug combination introduced for the treatment of solid tumors in the past 18 years. Clinical responses with this regimen were unprecedented

www.Dipex.org

September 26, 2003

Lyse was hospitalized today. She had been complaining of some shortness of breath, and a little difficulty breathing. I noticed that her belly was beginning to swell slightly.

Dr. Attas had examined Lyse and determined that she had fluid buildup in her left lung, likely caused by the tumor cells. It was always hard to tell with Lyse just how uncomfortable she was, or how much pain she was feeling. Her tolerance for physical and emotional discomfort was very high.

"Babe, you've got to tell me when you don't feel well, or when you think something is wrong. Please don't wait, or try to suffer through it. Tell me so we can get you the help you need, when you need it," I had scolded her. I was really mad that she had waited. From that point forward, I observed her closely for any subtle changes in her physical countenance.

I surmised that she knew, on some level, things were beginning to spiral out of control. Acknowledging and caving in to a new symptom perhaps meant deferring to the cancer.

Dr. Attas had instructed Lyse to get checked into the hospital right away. The fluid would be removed from her lung; afterward, she would receive her first treatment of GEMZAR.

Almost two liters of fluid were siphoned from Lyse's left lung. She said it felt good to take a deep breath again.

⤟

Our refrigerator was cloaked with magnetic souvenirs of our life together: a button from Pea Island Sanctuary on the Outer Banks, a Mickey Mouse button from Leo and Camille from their trip to Disney with the grandkids, pictures of Molly as a baby and pictures of the day we picked her up at the breeder, the list of cancer fighting foods from Holy Name Hospital, a small wood carving of a seagull and lighthouse from Block Island, Rhode Island, the number for the emergency animal clinic, and a scrap of paper Lyse had doodled on while talking on the phone one day shortly after she was diagnosed.

The scrap of doodle paper was roughly 3" x 3" in size. She had drawn on it with one of the assorted ballpoint pens we kept on the kitchen counter, next to the phone. The design included a mix of curvy lines, dots, tic-tac-toe boxes, and spirals. Together, they framed a concentrated blob of dark and deeply etched scribble—a blister of blackness fenced in by the surrounding, Escher-like sketches.

During dinner one night, I had glanced at the drawing on the refrigerator. I got up out of my chair to have a closer look.

"Babe, look at this," I said, and bent over to show her the artwork. "The really dark area in the middle is the cancer. It's surrounded by the lighter, brighter doodles—the white light. The white light isn't allowing the cancer to spread any further. It's keeping it contained and blotting it out. That's what comes to mind when I look at this picture."

"Hmm," she replied, nodding slowly, "I see what you're saying. That could be. It's definitely a hopeful way of looking at my mindless doodling."

"Well," I replied brightly, "I'm going to envision this when I do my imagery from now on."

I always felt that *my* fervor for Lyse's healing, and *my* passion and gusto for our combat, could inflame her to fight even harder. Just because someone isn't fighting as hard as you think they should, doesn't mean they're not fighting with everything they have, I later discerned.

Thursday, October 16, 2003

Lyse received a port today. She had undergone two additional infusions of GEMZAR this month before Dr. Attas advised her to see Dr. Freid for the port. The nurses were having trouble finding available veins in Lyse's arm for the IV. Some of the veins used previously had already collapsed and could not be used.

Breastcancer.org describes a port—or "port-a-cath"—as being about the size of a quarter, "but thick," and causing a bump under the skin. The port allows medication to flow directly into the "main blood supply entering the heart," which means the body receives the dose "quickly and efficiently."

By her fourth infusion of GEMZAR, on October 17, Lyse was relieved to not receive any more "sticks" in her arm. One, two, three, and the infusion was underway. It was uneventful.

⁊

Lyse didn't talk much about her illness. "How are you feeling?" was the unfailing start to every call. No matter what her state, Lyse's reply was the same: "I'm OK. Things are moving along."

Friends—except for Cathy and Joanne—colleagues, and family members—except Jeannine—didn't really know how ill she had begun to feel.

She craved the idle chatter of everyday life. She warmed to the latest news about her niece, Danielle, and her kids, her colleague, John, whom she mentored, her friend, Stephanie and her struggle with colon cancer, neighbor Dorothy and her aging Shih-Tzu, Cassie, Tara's school soccer meets, and Leo's ramblings about the quirky homeowners in Mill Brook Village.

She ached to know what substitute teachers were being called, how colleagues John and Michelle had made out in their new home, the latest about the trip to Atlantic City coworkers Judy and Etta had planned, and how Jeannine's husband Ron managed the radiation treatment for his prostate cancer.

During the past two months, Lyse had taken to letting the machine, or me, answer incoming calls. Most times, I could hardly bear to debrief callers, again and again.

I felt badly. People were only concerned. But I was angered, and exasperated by the plague of interruptions, and the need for others to know the details of our increasingly macabre existence.

Lyse thirsted for e-mail jokes, stories, and links to interesting web sites. She yearned for news from the outside, and tidbits from the lives of others. She craved the skinny on anyone but herself.

Cards and letters were, by far, the most appreciated and relished. Notes could be smiled at when the bouts of diarrhea had temporarily ceased. Written well-wishes could be savored when a meal couldn't be. Cards could be opened when there was no imminent threat of vomiting. The written word could restore a measure of control for one who was subjugated by a body blighted.

Tuesday, December 16, 2003

A CT scan was scheduled for Lyse today. She had received ten infusions of GEMZAR since September 26 and had been getting treatments on a weekly basis. I continued to be shocked at the insidious changes in her body that I noticed while she undressed each night. First, she slid off her button down blue cardigan, which was followed by the long-sleeved T-shirt. She removed her bra next, and then shed her blue, or black, Land's End sweat pants. She folded the warm and wrinkled garments, and then walked over to her dresser. She pulled out her sleep shirt—a short-sleeved tee such as the teal-green one she had worn while riding her Trek hybrid bicycle through northern New Jersey as part of Team Turtles, raising money for multiple sclerosis research, in 1995 and 1996.

Her belly had been slowly swelling while her arms and legs, mostly arms, were losing significant muscle mass. She appeared to be shrinking on top. Never bulky up top to begin with, her gaunt shoulders had now rolled inward; her breasts had deflated from meaty mammae to flopped party balloons pricked by a pin.

It was a grim thing happening to the body I had caressed and loved, and sidled up next to all hours of the night. I ached all over with pained sadness seeing my loved one trapped in a corpus I no longer recognized.

Sunday, December 28, 2003

Lyse had been running to the bathroom with bouts of diarrhea. It came fast, often faster than she could sprint. She began wearing the special underwear as backup, for the times she didn't quite make it. She lost her appetite, also. She stopped drinking the occasional half-glass of wine altogether. She said she didn't have a taste for it anymore.

We had become wine connoisseurs-in-the-making during our time together. Our favorite was Chardonnay, preferably the buttery, vanilla laced kind, with a touch of oak and mild tannins. We indulged ourselves with varietals from Napa Valley, Oregon, Australia and New Zealand. Our pleasure was lounging on the couch for thirty minutes each night, before dinner, sipping Chardonnay, and bantering about the day. Sue Simmons and Chuck Scarborough from NBC, channel 4, delivered the news in the background.

Wine shopping was one of our greatest pleasures. Total Wine, a supermarket-type store down the street, was chock-full of wines and micro-brewed beers from around the world, specialty candies, crackers and nuts. We'd spend a couple of hours reading labels on bottles of Merlot, Pinot Noir, blends, Cabs, and Chardonnay, picking our stock carefully. Our cart brimmed with libations bursting with hearty flavors of berry, pepper, chocolate, vanilla, citrus and oak.

In the spring and summer, cocktail hour would unfold on the deck, with Molly at our feet. We would languish on the faded wood-turned-gray Adirondack chairs. Often, neighbors walking their dogs, would call up to us. Stewart, with his Shih-Tzu, Mindy, Debbie, and her horse-like chocolate Lab, Simba, or Dorothy, with her frail and rotund Cassie.

Stewart developed colon cancer shortly before Lyse was diagnosed. He endured his own battle with surgery and debilitating follow-up radiation. Early on, in Lyse's illness, we had returned from chemotherapy, and were both making our way up the driveway toward the house. Lyse caught sight of Stewart out in his front yard with Mindy. She waved, and then turned around. She lumbered slowly over toward his house, to see how he was doing. She was often groggy and a little muddled after her infusions. He saw her coming, and began walking down the street to meet her halfway.

I was beholden to the cinematography of the moment. I was witness to a snapshot in time that held such distinction, that was so supreme, I believe I saw the clouds part to reveal a ray of heavenly light; trumpets of angels cantillated the goodwill of men toward each other.

Two frail souls, pale and thin of hair, each riddled with the scourge of cells gone corrupt, greeted each other knowingly, with shared experiences, and collective grief and loss. They embraced each other in the street, communing during the battle, reciprocating unspoken sadness, and proud to have come this far, anyway.

My focus on them, I cried before I realized I was doing so.

❦

The quilt on our brass double bed was a hand fashioned patchwork of soothing blue, pink, cream, and sage stripes, solids and florals. The package from L.L. Bean arrived two days after we had ordered it, in late 2002, before Lyse got sick.

The quilt's colors were highlighted by the lusciously soft muted pink sheets we bought with it. We excitedly dressed the bed with the new furnishings. The combination was peerlessly pretty.

Our $320.00 investment cocooned us each night in cottony snugness, lulling us to sleep, caressing our limbs as we shifted in our dreams.

All of our investments were only what we needed, and nothing more. What we did buy was of quality. Spending on incidentals, or things that would serve no real purpose in our lives, seemed foolish.

It wasn't long before the ravages of the cancer began leaving their mark on just about everything in the house, including our beloved coverlet. The Lexapro curbed my *frenzied* need to clean and get everything in order *immediately*, but it didn't curb my need *to do it*. My desire to maintain order and symmetry was only slightly relaxed, no longer a burning mania.

Still, I came undone by the soiled quilt. I removed it, and drove immediately to the dry cleaner. I replaced it with an old comforter that could easily be washed when necessary. I was overwrought and agitated, not at Lyse, but because the quilt was no longer on the bed—because the old, less attractive quilt was now on the bed. Because the old quilt upset my balance of what was and should be in the bedroom. I was angry at the OCD for making it seem like I was angry with Lyse.

Wednesday, January 21, 2004

Lyse's infusions of GEMZAR continued on a weekly basis. Recently, we'd made runs to the emergency room. Fairly consistent diarrhea and vomiting had caused Lyse to become dehydrated. She was spending more time sitting on the couch, and demonstrated very little initiative or energy for undertaking activities of daily living—such as showering or clipping her nails. Preparing even simple snacks had become a chore.

We were about to climb into bed that evening, when Lyse asked me to look at something on her leg.

"Do you think I should call Dr. Attas about this tomorrow morning?" she asked me, pointing to the calf of her right leg.

I could see that her right leg, from the knee down, was remarkably swollen. I ran a cupped hand gently over the area, and then did the same on her left leg. I was alarmed.

"Tomorrow morning?" I asked calmly, but sternly. "Babe, I'm not sure what this is, but my hunch is this swelling is due to something going on. We really need to go to the emergency room tonight and have this looked at. We shouldn't wait at all."

I had been craving bedtime since I came home from work. I was particularly worn out that day and longed for some mindless TV time and deep slumber.

"Come, sweetie," I prodded, "let's get dressed. I'll pack you a bag, and we'll head over to the hospital."

Thirty minutes later, we were being examined by the emergency room doctor. Sixty minutes after that, Lyse was admitted for a blood clot the length of her right leg. She stayed in the hospital for one week until the clot had dissipated. She remained on Coumadin—a blood thinner—as a preventative measure.

We understood from the doctor that the blood clot, had it dislodged, would have meant certain and immediate death for Lyse. I wondered, after all was said and done, if that scenario wouldn't have been the merciful one.

✍

Sidney had offered me his stepfatherly wisdom many times throughout the years. This time was no different.

His insight into human nature and all of its foibles was garnered from his own gritty life experiences as well as those of his patients.

January 27, 2004

Hi Cher,

Mom related to me some of the new, added difficulties you girls are experiencing. If I may, I would like to contribute some thoughts. I am older than she, and have seen a little more of these situations in my lifetime, professionally and otherwise.

I think that your continued functioning as breadwinner and household manager is a prime necessity. If, God forbid, your health suffers and/or you lose your job, you will both be in very deep yogurt indeed. Your continued capability to pursue your career and the other important things in your life must remain intact and solid. I don't think you can do all the schlepping, nursing care at home, medical liaison work, dog stuff, hospital vigils, etc. etc. and still keep your head above water.

In my opinion, the situation urgently demands additional manpower, and the other members of Lyse's family must contribute – either by personal attendance at your home, doctor visits, hospital when necessary, etc., or by substantial cash contributions to underwrite outside hired help. "Homemaking" services are readily available commercially, LPN care if needed, commercial pickup and delivery of patients for medical appointments, etc. are available here, and I presume they are there also.

You absolutely cannot carry a full time management-level job with its attendant responsibilities, and then do full time patient-care and household management at home. If you do, I am afraid that you will fold. It appears that you have a sick girl on your hands, and you must demand help from the other members of the family. This is a bad chronic progressive sickness you are dealing with. You must call increasingly on family and/or community support. You may have to do the quarterbacking and managerial things, but other people will have to do the day-to-day supportive tasks in the trenches.

Take care of yourself. We don't want this to destroy you emotionally, physically, or financially.

If I can help in any more direct way, or discuss this further, don't hesitate.

Love,
Sidney

Friday, January 30, 2004

Dr. Attas had advised that treatment with GEMZAR was to be discontinued. He would start Lyse on Topotecan right away.

Topotecan is one of the newer chemotherapy drugs, and has been around, and in use for some years. It is a synthetic product, very similar to a natural compound, Camptothecin, which was driven [sic] from a Chinese tree, "Camptotheca acuminate".

Topotecan is normally given by intravenous infusion over 30 minutes, daily for five consecutive days.

www.tirgan.com

According to the topotecan.com web site, it is "used to treat advanced cervical and ovarian cancers as well as small cell lung cancer that has continued to grow after first line therapy." The drug works by "stopping the growth of cancer cells by preventing the development of elements necessary for cell division."

Sunday, February 1, 2004

Monique arrived today. She'll stay with us for as long as we need her. It will be three months.

Michelle and Danielle, two of Monique's three daughter, had driven their mom to our house. It was a three-and-a-half hour trip from Providence,

Rhode Island. They showed up at our door laden with suitcases, oversized totes, and grocery sacks.

We were relieved to see her and the help she represented, the sharing of a burden too great for the two of us anymore. I helped the Caseys bring in the load of satchels from Danielle's burgundy mini-van.

All bags, except those with food, were plopped in the foyer. I offered to take all groceries into the kitchen, where I hurriedly began to stock the freezer, fridge and cabinets. I was feeling invaded. The fragile order I had managed to retain during the past seventeen months was being threatened again—this time by people who were here to help us, and make our lives easier. I had to get everything put away, neatly, and then I would feel better. I tossed the empty bags, and took Monique's suitcases upstairs. Then, I relaxed a little.

Monique, Michelle, Danielle, and Lyse made their way into the living room to sit down. I heard the couch squeak as Michelle, Monique's oldest, and largest-of-girth daughter, sat down. I cringed, thinking maybe a spring had popped.

Every benign, naive movement by a visitor in our home generated a powerful, visceral response. My need to control behaviors that might effect a mess needing to be cleaned, extended to those entering our home as well, but not in a way apparent to the visitors. It was important to me and Lyse that all houseguests felt completely at ease and fully welcomed. Our home was a haven for us; we wanted to extend that tranquility to those we loved.

The Lexapro enabled me to temporarily overlook the insignia of the visitor—the dirty glass on the coffee table, the drop of urine on the toilet seat, the crooked bathroom rug, the specks of dirt on the carpet, the crumbs on the wood floor—and to right things when that person wasn't looking.

My response was a silent one, known only to me, and felt only by me. Innate and powerful, it gripped the sinew of my neck and shoulders, pinched the flesh of my abdomen, strangled the rhythmic in and out of my diaphragm, and clenched my jaw together in a seizing motion.

Only later, when I could put things back the way they were, did I get relief.

"I made beef stew, chicken casseroles, and vegetable soup," I heard Danielle announce to her "Tante Lyse."

Danielle had attended the College of Culinary Arts at Johnson and Wales University, in Providence, Rhode Island. She was a gifted chef and enjoyed creating dishes for friends and family.

I stacked the frozen items neatly in the freezer, according to entrée type. Danielle had packaged the soups in round containers, and the casseroles and stews in square tubs. I had to move our frozen Omaha steak filets down a shelf, plus take them out of the box, but everything fit well. I was pleased.

Next, I unpacked the grocery bags of dry goods and food in boxes, cans and cartons. Monique enjoyed carbohydrate rich foods like pasta and crackers. Unlike Jeannine, her diet was light in fresh fruits and vegetables. I pulled out a box of Chicken in the Basket crackers and glared at the contents label. High in fat, salt and carbs.

I don't want Lyse eating these, especially now.

Monique, for all of her years eating only a moderately healthy diet, was extremely healthy, robust and energetic. She looked at least ten years younger than her age. She had encountered no major medical problems except arthritis, which was beginning to become very painful.

How is it that some people are just predisposed to a clean bill of health in spite of a so-so diet? How is it that Lyse, for all of her healthy eating, vitamin popping ways, could be sitting here battling such a vicious disease?

The absurdity of it all angered me. I pulled out four boxes of Kraft Mac and Cheese.

Good. Chemical cheese and pasty pasta with no known nutrients.

Canned peas, tomatoes, and corn, chocolate chip cookies, white bread hoagie rolls, Velveeta cheese and Ritz crackers followed. I glumly maneuvered the items into the pantry, shaking my head and sighing.

Monique can eat this if she wants to, but it's no good for Lyse.

❧

We ate dinner together every night, in the beginning. Monique prepared ground beef with canned tomatoes and shell pasta—the Caseys called it American chop suey—as well as macaroni and cheese, breaded chicken cutlets and spaghetti with sauce from a jar. We also enjoyed Danielle's home-cooked dinners. I'd make salads to go with the meals. We sat at the dining room table. Monique and I took pleasure in the wine we shared.

One weekend morning, shortly after Monique's arrival, I began to prepare a mid-morning snack of date nut bread and cream cheese. Lyse and Monique were chatting quietly in the living room. I called to them, and asked if they wanted to join me. By the time they arrived, I had amassed a small, but contained pile of crumbs on the kitchen counter, ready to be taken to the sink. I had my back turned to them while I smeared the pieces of dark, nutty bread with the cream cheese. When I turned around to carry the plates to the table, I saw Monique sweeping the pile of crumbs into her palm.

That's really nice of her to clean up my mess. It's so considerate, and helpful. She must notice me freaking out over the chaos in the house. I stopped abruptly, mid-way between counter and table, caught in my tracks by the sight of Monique clapping and rubbing her palms together over the floor. I looked down and saw the chunky, dark crumbs scattered over a wide swath of tiles. I remember it now as I saw it then—all in slow motion. I remember my gasp, and Lyse's wide eyes. I remember not being able to stop myself from running for the Dust Buster. When the crumbs had been sucked up, we all sat down for our snack. A rather innocent act had the power to undo me so completely. It had me in its grip. I wasn't able to hide my response, nor could I wait to vacuum in private.

Much, much later, Lyse and I managed to laugh about it.

Whereas Lyse and Jeannine had a place for everything, Monique was more relaxed. For her extended stay, she filled her tote bags with sketch paper, charcoal pencils, oil paints, eight to ten books, sweaters, a blanket, and old photos to share with Lyse.

We set up her bunk in the spare bedroom, which was also our office and contained my desk. Soon, bags and belongings were sprawled out all over the floor and on the bed. It looked like an artist's bohemian studio, without the easel. I did okay as long as I didn't look in the room. When I had to use the desk, I crept gingerly through the maze, reflexively patting piles and stealthily coercing Monique's belongings into some kind of symmetrical scheme I could tolerate while in there.

Monique brought new life to the house—a breath of fresh air. She made us laugh with boisterous stories of her audacious ways in high school. We sat at the table after dinner talking about the family, or neighbours from Lyse's old

Providence neighborhood from when she was a kid. Lyse savored the banter and Monique's lighthearted, optimistic demeanor.

Monique's nurturing and coddling manner actually helped both of us. We were in need of her comforting ways, for very different reasons, by the time she joined our household.

Lyse received chemo infusions five days a week, every third week, beginning Monday, February 2. It was around this time that the diarrhea began to occur on a daily basis. About a week later, the vomiting followed suit. She couldn't keep much down. One night, she vomited her spaghetti right back up into her plate at the dining room table.

Monique fixed her small meals—a cup of yogurt, a soft-boiled egg on toast, a mug of soup—but most of them either came back up or went right through her. She took Compazine to control the nausea and vomiting as needed. This series of sad and unfortunate events continued into March.

Evident during the latter part of February was a subtle change in Lyse's social connection to others. She rarely initiated a phone call, mostly because she didn't feel well enough to sustain a conversation.

I later learned that it is not uncommon for the terminally ill patient to begin disconnecting socially from his/her world anywhere from one to three months before passing. It is a preparation, of sorts, for the time of transition.

Wednesday, March 31, 2004

Lyse had a CT scan today. Dr. Attas wanted to gauge the success of the Topotecan. We remained hopeful on the surface, but deep down, I think all three of us knew that things were probably not in our favor.

Friday, April 2, 2004

Lyse's last entry in her Yorkie calendar was marked with the appointment, "Dr. Attas 11:45."

He gave us the results of Lyse's most recent CT scan. She had a "small bowel to large bowel obstruction." He said surgery could be done to remove the mass. He told us that to give Lyse more drugs at this time "doesn't make sense."

He wasn't certain if the bowel obstruction was due to surgery, or a mass. He sent Lyse for an x-ray to make that determination. He admitted her to the hospital immediately.

Sunday, April 4, 2004

Lyse underwent surgery today to remove the bowel obstruction. Dr. George Christoudias performed the operation. I found him to be very passionate and approachable. Monique and I waited for Lyse to be returned to her room. He updated us late that afternoon before Lyse got back.

"During surgery, we found bilateral pleural effusions," he began.

He explained that "pleural" had to do with the fluid in the lining of the lung. As described by the National Lung Health Education Program web site, nlhep.org, "pleural effusions occur when the rate of fluid formation exceeds that of fluid absorption."

He went on to tell us that he had removed Lyse's colon, as the malignant cells were found "stuck to her bowel." He also told us that there were malignant cells "all over the abdomen."

Monique and I looked at each other and couldn't speak, for our despair.

"It is time for hospice," Dr. Christoudias stated sadly. He looked at us and then lowered his eyes toward the floor.

CHAPTER EIGHT:
IT IS WHAT IT IS

"I didn't say anything about hospice!" Dr. Attas bellowed into the phone.

His shockingly loud words pierced my eardrum.

"I'm Lyse's oncologist and I call all the shots—no one else!"

His unrestrained barking might have been a precursor for a knockdown.

I stood in the hospital corridor, a few doors down from Lyse's room. I had called him right after speaking to Dr. Christoudias. I was impaled on his words, and berated by his tone. My already weakened constitution now felt like a saltine under a bulldozer.

He continued roaring, "We still have more options! It's not over yet!"

"But Dr. Christoudias said…" I began.

"I decide if and when it's time for hospice, no one else!" he butted in.

"All right, then, Dr. Attas," I replied, my calm voice betraying the fact that my insides felt hacked.

"If you have experimental drugs in mind as the next step, I do know that Lyse has already said she's not interested in those," I stated matter-of-factly.

Lyse had been very clear, all along, that she didn't want drugs that were still being tested. "There are some very good experimental drugs being used right now," he continued, his tone firm and not as harsh.

"I will get in touch with you and Lyse to talk about those options," he told me next, and then promptly hung up.

"OK, thank you, Dr. Attas," I said. The buzz of the dial tone was the only sound coming from the other end of the line.

Monique was gracious about my role as manager of Lyse's legal, medical and financial matters. I made sure the hospital *and* nurse's station had copies of Lyse's living will, which contained medical directives, health care power of attorney, and general power of attorney. All of these legal documents invoked me as the person, named by Lyse, who would execute legal and medical decisions should she be unable to. Some of the duties I had agreed to, on her behalf, included: continuing or terminating health care, withholding or withdrawing artificially administered food and fluids for life-sustaining measures, and authorizing treatment for "maximum comfort and freedom from pain."

Lyse was returned to her room shortly after I finished speaking with Dr. Attas. She now had a colostomy bag—a pouch on the outside of the body that collected waste directly from the intestine.

She was on pain medication for the incision, but she was awake and aware. Monique and I agreed that we both should be present when I spoke with her about the results of the surgery.

❧

Dr. Attas never spoke to us about the experimental drugs. He knew what Lyse's feelings were about not using them. Although they were our only remaining option, it was clear we really didn't have any options left.

❧

Monique sat on the right side of Lyse's bed, and I sat on the left. I didn't sit, actually. I stood up, and then bent over so I was face-to-face with Lyse. This was too important a conversation for me to not stand. Monique stood, also. We took Lyse's hands in ours.

"Babe," I began, the skin on the nape of my neck tingling, the tingling creeping slowly upward onto the base of my skull, crawling higher until it ceased somewhere near the crown of my head.

I felt a strange heat dilate my groin. A weakness numbed my legs, and my lungs seemed choked of air.

My voice was curiously calm, and assured.

"Dr. Christoudias gave us the results of your surgery. The cancer had spread to your bowel and was causing a blockage."

I stopped to breath, and swallowed a large glob of saliva.

"He had to remove a part of your intestine to clear the blockage. There is still a lot of cancer left behind that can't be removed, because it's stuck to your abdomen," I continued, slowly, and matter-of-factly, as if I were giving a presentation at work.

"He believes, based on what he saw during surgery, that there is nothing more that can be done to get rid of the cancer," I continued gently. "I spoke with

Dr. Attas earlier, and he said we could try experimental drugs next, but that is our only choice right now," I said, slowly blinking and swallowing hard.

Lyse shook her head as I said "experimental drugs." I wasn't surprised, even at that dire point in time.

Thursday, April 8, 2004

We sang "Happy Birthday" to Lyse this afternoon. She had turned sixty-three. Monique bought a muffin at the hospital cafeteria and stuck a red candle in it. It was one of those moments you see in a movie that causes you to spill large, hot tears into your bucket of greasy popcorn. Except we weren't at the movie; we were in it. When you're in the movie, you need to act according to the script. Emotions might just take you off task and compromise the job at hand.

Thursday, April 15, 2004

Lyse's condition, post-bowel surgery, was considered "subacute" by the hospital and Blue Cross Blue Shield of New Jersey. As defined by the National Association of Subacute / Post Acute Care: "…Subacute care is a comprehensive, cost-effective in-patient level of care for patients who: have had an acute event resulting from injury, illness or exacerbation of a disease process; have a determined course of treatment; though stable, require diagnostics or invasive procedures, but not intensive procedures requiring an acute level of care."

I learned this from Carol, a social worker from Holy Name's social services department. Carol was empathetic and kind, and said she knew the level of pain and sadness I must be feeling. Her phone kept ringing at the little counter she shared with two other social workers, in a cramped room next to the nurse's station. Fatigue stung my eyes; anguish needled my heart. Hope was a long forgotten friend.

Carol said the next level of care for Lyse, beginning today, would be "in-patient hospice." She also told me that she had already spoken with BCBS on our behalf, and that the insurance company would only pay for ten days of in-patient hospice.

Lyse has ten days to die or else. Is that what they're telling me?

Carol explained that after ten days, I would need to bring Lyse home, or pay for room and board out-of-pocket.

"Of course, I want to bring her home," I explained. "I've already contacted the medical supply place for a bed," I continued.

It was inconceivable that I *not* bring Lyse home for her final days. I envisioned placing the bed in the living room, facing the deck, so she could watch her birds outside the sliding glass doors. She used to zoom in on the little birds with the "backyard binoculars" I had bought her at L.L. Bean. Molly could sit on her bed and give her kisses.

Monique and I could turn her, bathe her, and manage the IV drip. We'd be visited by hospice and could always call in a part-time aide to help us where necessary. We would do what needed to be done.

The medications Lyse received intravenously, during this time, were Dilantin, Ativan, and Zofran. The pharmaceuticals were introduced as a means of "keeping her comfortable," and nothing more.

The National Institute of Neurological Disorders and Stroke reports that "cancers and benign tumors can infiltrate or exert damaging pressure on nerve fibers."

Dilantin is used for cancer patients to help alleviate peripheral neuropathy. Peripheral neuropathy, according to the NINDS, can be rooted in physical injury, systemic disease, and autoimmune disorders.

Peripheral neuropathy is described by the NINDS as: "…damage to the peripheral nervous system, the vast communications network that transmits information from the brain and spinal cord (the central nervous system) to every other part of the body. Peripheral nerves also send sensory information back to the brain and spinal cord, such as a message that the feet are cold or a finger is burned. Damage to the peripheral nervous system interferes with these vital connections."

∽

We would dance, in the living room, to *Always*, sung by Ella Fitzgerald. We'd hold Molly for a verse or two, and sing softly the whole way through.

I'll be loving you always
With a love that's true always… (excerpt)

Written by Irving Berlin

So many times we said to each other that our love was forever, would last forever, and would be forever. Ours was a connection that transcended words, even the limits of the earth and sky. We had arrived into this life already linked. Our partnership had played out before, in other lives, other times, and in different bodies and genders. It didn't matter what it was before or what it had been this time. Each soul of the whole recognizes the other, and it just is. The props of life— home, car, work, stuff—become accessories to the main event. It is our own love story that is told over and over again. It is the story of unconditional giving and receiving, perhaps the greatest reason for coming here at all.

Saturday, April 17, 2004

The head nurse in charge of Lyse's care spoke with me about a Do Not Resuscitate (DNR) order. Familydoctor.org describes this as follows:

A do not resuscitate (DNR) order is another kind of advance directive. A DNR is a request not to have cardiopulmonary resuscitation (CPR) if your heart stops or if you stop breathing. (Unless given other instructions, hospital staff will try to help all patients whose heart has stopped or who have stopped breathing.) You can use an advance directive form or tell your doctor that you don't want to be resuscitated. In this case, a DNR order is put in your medical chart by your doctor. DNR orders are accepted by doctors and hospitals in all states.

I was asked if I wanted the order added to Lyse's chart. I knew what her wishes were. I knew the answer was "yes."

A peculiar prickling snaked its way up the back of my neck, what I had felt the day we spoke with Lyse about hospice. I was in uncharted territory. The sensation was a primal one. I recognized it as something not called upon often. It was something that rested deep within my DNA—an ancient coping mechanism handed down biologically through the centuries. The responsibility of it was leviathan; the honor even more so. Here they were, the end-of-life "what ifs" we had talked about over pasta and red wine, staring us in the face, budging not an inch.

We had prepared. We were doing the best we could.

✖

Ron and Jeannine drove up from Florida shortly after Lyse's surgery. Since November, they had been wintering at their home in Port St. Lucie. Ron continued home to Massachusetts; Jeannine would stay until the end.

Monique had been sleeping at the hospital since Lyse was admitted. Jeannine would do the same.

Thus began the vigil.

Sunday, April 18, 2004

I hadn't gone to work since Lyse's surgery, when it was clear Lyse had very little time left. Mike in human resources asked that I submit a Family Medical Leave form, to be signed by Lyse's physician. I met with Nice, and she helped me complete the paperwork. I mailed it the same day.

✖

Lyse was awake on and off throughout the day. She was fairly alert, though sleepy from the medication. Jeannine applied cream to her hands and arms, laid cool washcloths on her forehead, and dabbed Vaseline on her increasingly cracked lips.

Jeannine had brought a few old family photos she had at the house in Florida. She placed a faded brown and white picture on Lyse's bed table—Lyse and Monique posing in plaid dresses, Lyse the big sister holding Monique's hand— and encouraged Lyse to look at the snapshot.

"Remember, Lyse?" Jeannine asked. "You and Monique on the front lawn in Providence. You two were such good friends. You were the big sister," she cooed, making eye contact with Lyse. "That's right, you were."

Lyse's eyes followed Jeannine's gestures. She listened intently but did not speak. She seemed too tired for that. Her eyes disclosed sadness and frustration. I was pained to see it.

I took her hand in mine and sensed the ebbing life. The warmth, strength and softness I was accustomed to was no longer there. I kissed her on the forehead.

"You know how much I love you, babe, don't you?" I said softly.

She look at me and nodded once. Her eyes were moist.

∽

At night, Jeannine and Monique took turns sleeping in the lounge at the end of the hallway, across from Lyse's room. One sat with Lyse while the other slept.

We were all there during the day. I'd visit from early morning until mid-afternoon and go back home for a walk with Molly, a quick nap, and a light supper. Then, I'd return to the hospital to stay from dinnertime until 8:30 p.m.

Intuitively, I began to carve out small breathers for myself. My afternoon naps at home sustained me for evening visits. My walks with Molly gave me the juice to collaborate with the nurses, and the efficacy to sort things through with Jeannine and Monique.

The support of Cathy and Joanne for doctor visits and taking Lyse to treatments had been critical to me keeping it all together, barely.

Beginning with Lyse's initial surgery in 2002, I had been a racehorse, charging out of the gate full force. However, as Sidney had pointed out, the caregiver also needs care.

One morning, shortly after I had arrived at the hospital, Monique approached me. She asked if we could talk in the family lounge. Jeannine was sitting in Lyse's room.

"Jeannine and I spoke about the cremation. You know, Catholics don't believe in cremation, although we know this is Lyse's wish. We were thinking we'd love to have a service for the family up in Rhode Island, and thought it would be nice to bury Lyse's body next to Georgette, instead of having her cremated and sprinkled somewhere. We may not be able to bury her in the cemetery at the church if she is cremated. There are so many people from the family and neighborhood who knew and loved Lyse and would want to pay their respects. I know the plans are in writing, but we were hoping it might be something you would consider." She spoke with consternation, wringing her hands and furrowing her brow.

"I want you to spread my ashes somewhere special to the two of us," I could hear Lyse saying to me, years earlier.

Conflict. Negotiation. Resolution. I can do this.

I took a deep breath but it ratcheted out of me, and punctured on the sharp edges of nerves, stress, and fatigue.

"I understand the concerns you and Jeannine have. I do know that Lyse wants to be cremated and be put to rest in a place special to the two of us," I stated.

She looked so sad and sorrowful. I wanted the family to be at peace, and to also have a resolution. The kind of remains and type of burial somehow seemed trivial, compared to the suffering and agony we all were enduring at the time, especially Lyse. Still, a problem was a thing that needed a resolution. So, I mistakenly took on their thorny burden and proceeded to help them fix it.

I still squirm when I think about what I did next. I'm haunted by it and expect I will be always. I've historically been a fixer—never afraid to face a problem head on. And, to a fault, I sometimes didn't think about what problem belonged to me, and what problem didn't. Often, it was more important just to get the problem fixed. I still wonder if the good I did for Lyse was eclipsed by my blunder.

Lyse was awake, and smiled faintly when I walked into her room.

"How are you doing, sweetie?" I asked, smiling and kissing her on the lips.

Her dry lips parted into a faint smile. She mumbled, "Okay."

"Babe, Monique and Jeannine would really like you to be buried next to Georgette. They want you to be close to the family." I heard myself talking and felt disconnected from the source of the words.

"I know you want me to put you at rest in a place special to the two of us," I continued, feeling lightheaded and floaty. "Sweetie, I want to do what you're comfortable with. I know how important Jeannine and Monique are to you. I wanted you to know their wishes," I went on, my insides wriggling. "I will do what you want me to," I finished, looking at her sadly.

She took a breath and said, "Just do what is comfortable for everyone." Then, she closed her eyes to rest a while.

"I just want to do the right thing for you, babe," I replied. "I love you so much, sweetie."

I kissed her again and then walked softly out of the room.

Looking back now, I believe that exchange, although painful for me, may have actually been a blessing for her. Up until the end, then, I was keeping her deeply involved in my decisions, seeking her input, and most importantly, garnering her as an active participant in our partnership. Just as it had always been.

❧

Monique came up to me later that day and said she and Jeannine had decided they were comfortable with, and resolved about, Lyse being cremated, since that was her wish.

"Would you consider having her buried next to Georgette in Providence?" Monique asked hopefully.

I knew how much Georgette meant to Lyse. I also knew how important this was to the family. I understood how important Jeannine and Monique were to Lyse.

"That would be fine," I replied softly. "I think everyone would be comfortable with that."

Monique smiled and hugged me tightly. She was beaming with relief and gratification.

April 20, 2004

I met with Carol from social services today. She told me that effective April 25, in-hospital hospice would no longer be paid for by Lyse's insurance company. I needed to make some decisions soon so that Lyse would have a place to go, come that day.

"You have five possible options," Carol began, concern and earnestness emanating in her face, audible in her voice.

"You can bring Lyse home and hire a live-in nurse, if you feel you can't manage the turning, medication, suctioning, catheter, oxygen, etc., duties that will be necessary for you to perform. A live-in nurse will cost approximately a thousand dollars per week," she stated.

"If Lyse's death seems imminent at that time, there may be a chance that insurance will pay for an extended in-hospital hospice," she continued.

"You also have the option of placing Lyse in Cavalry Hospital, in the Bronx. This is a hospital that cares for patients with advanced cancer and provides 'palliative care,' which means that the patient's symptoms are managed and treated, not the disease. The goal is to keep the patient as comfortable as possible," she continued.

The in-hospital hospice social workers, Marge and Charlene, had talked to Lyse and me, a few days before, about Calvary as an option. Lyse was very clear that she didn't want to spend her last days at Calvary.

"I already know that Lyse doesn't want to go to Calvary," I replied.

"You can also keep Lyse here, in the hospital's hospice program, and pay for services out-of-pocket. As a last possible option, we may be able to get Lyse transferred back as a critical care patient, but I need to check into that first," she concluded.

I had been taking notes as she spoke, and looked up when she finished. I was at a loss for words.

"I know it's a lot right now," she offered gently. "For now, just think about what you might like to do and we'll talk some more later on."

"I really want to bring her home, but I'm just not sure we can handle everything, medically, that needs to be done. I could consider hiring a nurse, then," I responded, looking at her. "I believe that is what I would like to do."

I thanked her for her time, and her very thorough explanation of everything. All the phones on her little desk were ringing shrilly. They contrasted sharply with the quiet hum of the hallway. I made my way back to Lyse's room to visit some more.

Lyse had been receiving nutrition through total parenteral therapy (TPN). According to doctoronline.nhs.uk, "parenteral" means "administered any other way except by the mouth." This was a way of feeding a patient intravenously when complications such as intestinal surgery, vomiting, or diarrhea prevented the patient from ingesting and digesting food in a normal manner. A tube was placed into one of the large veins, like under the collarbone. Feeding could take several hours per day.

Lyse also had a drip for pain medication, a catheter for urination, and an oxygen clip. Jeannine had taken to rubbing ice on her lips so she could feel the cooling wetness. Jeannine was also beginning to suction the mucous that was building up in Lyse's mouth.

Lyse was sleeping a good deal, around the clock. She awakened now and then to look around the room, or to gaze at us. She seemed not to really focus on anything. Rather, her eyes just wandered a bit, and then she would stare. She groaned from time to time. Jeannine interpreted this as pain and asked me to ask the nurse for another dose of medication. For the most part, fortunately, she seemed to be pain-free. The nurses were responsive, gentle, and benevolent.

Jeannine and Monique took turns going down to the cafeteria for snacks. I brought sandwiches and fruit for them from home, also. They had been sponge-bathing and making due with a few items of clothing. Their bedside watch continued quietly, and fervently. They were the sentinels. Lyse would have no other.

⤐

I contacted Father George from St. Peter's Catholic Church in River Edge, and asked if he would consider officiating at Lyse's service. Lyse and I didn't know him, but he came highly recommended from Bridie. She had gone to St. Peter's for years.

Wednesday, April 21, 2004

Dr. Attas stopped into Lyse's room today. He greeted me cordially, stood barely inside the door, glanced at Lyse, and lifted his arm to her in what seemed to be a combination of waves and salutes.

"Hey there, Lyse," he called over to her. "You doing all right?"

He looked around the room, said terse hellos to Monique and Jeannine, and shuffled his feet in place.

His breathing was loud and snorty almost. He fidgeted.

"Well, you hang in there, Lyse, now," he called to her.

He looked at all of us, said good-bye, turned on his heels, and walked out. I heard the soft clop-clop of his clogs as he made his way down the hallway.

❧

I understood Dr. Attas's retort to Lyse's impending death. We are all entitled to respond in our own way. Dr. Attas cared so much for Lyse, that it pained him to see his treatments, his medical plan, and his intentions for her, fail in the face of a few noxious cells.

He couldn't save her. He wanted nothing more than to do so. It had become the opposite of an artist standing back and admiring his work. The bucket of paint had spilled and desecrated the carefully rendered life he had worked so painstakingly to restore.

Sunday, April 25, 2004
Morning

Lyse had been in a coma for two days now. Jeannine and the nurses insisted that her time was close, by a day or two, if not hours. Jeannine had been watching Lyse's urine output, which had turned orange, from a dark yellow. She said you could gauge death by the output of the kidneys.

She continued to suction Lyse's mouth, wiped her brow with a damp washcloth, and applied Vaseline to her lips.

Lyse was sleeping deeply now. Her breathing was barely audible; the rise and fall of her chest was hardly discernable. It seemed as though each breath would be her last. I focused on the white light, surrounded her with peace and calm, and told her it was OK to let go.

The mucousy rattle of her breathing made my head and neck muscles taut. I thought I couldn't bear this excruciating loitering of life, this life-shadow that lingered and defied the sun that tried to extinguish it.

I caught my breath and held it, for the strain of it all.

Sunday, April 25, 2004

Late afternoon

I had taken a nap. Molly and I had just returned from our walk, and I was warming up leftover pasta fagioli soup in the microwave. I was famished. My glass of Chardonnay sat at the kitchen table. My placemat was set with a napkin and spoon. My bread and butter laid neatly on the plate.

I was rushing a bit, so I could get back to the hospital.

Ring. Ring.

I saw Monique's cell phone number on the display.

"Hi, Monique," I said, after picking up the phone.

"Are you eating?" she asked. Her apprehension was palpable.

"Yes. I'll be finished shortly," I replied, with my heart quickening.

"Hurry," she said quietly.

"I'm on my way," I replied and hung up.

I gulped three spoonfuls of soup, put the bowl in the fridge, ran Molly up to the bedroom, grabbed my bag, and headed out the door. I screeched out of the driveway and headed toward Route 4. The highway just might get me there faster. Heart pounding and temples throbbing, I floored it, dodging around cars in my way. I whipped off the exit and drove one mile south on Teaneck Road. I turned into the hospital, and took the first visitor's spot I saw. I sprinted through the automatic doors of the front entrance and flew past the welcome desk.

"I have to get upstairs right away," I gasped, racing past the astonished gray-haired volunteer ladies.

I knew, during the ride up in the elevator. I felt her leave, as the elevator climbed through the floors. I perceived her transition as the elevator buzzer announced our arrival.

Running down the hallway past the nurse's desk, I breezed into Lyse's room.

Jeannine was whimpering, bent down on her knees, and leaning over Lyse. She was stroking Lyse's hair. Monique stood silently at the foot of the bed. Jeannine got up so I could see Lyse. A sob sprang forth from the abyss of my person. I knelt down and rested my forehead on Lyse's abdomen, and felt the warmth of her body quickly dissipating. I cradled her right hand in mine. It, too, was succumbing to the coldness of death.

I placed a lingering kiss on her forehead, and I murmured, "You are mine. I am yours. Always."

Tuesday, July 13, 1999

Molly raced around the backyard in a big circle, while Lyse and I chased her. The sun was close to setting on this radiant evening. The warm breeze ruffled Molly's black puppy fur, and set a glow over Lyse's head of brilliant silver hair. Our townhouse stood behind us, along with two Adirondack chairs still warm from the flush of a robust summer sun.

The grass, bright green under Molly's paws, and our feet, was cool and luscious. Round and round we went, laughing, screeching and gasping for air, lost in our otherworld, joy unbounded, enchantment discovered, and bliss cultivated.

This is what I remember.

THE END

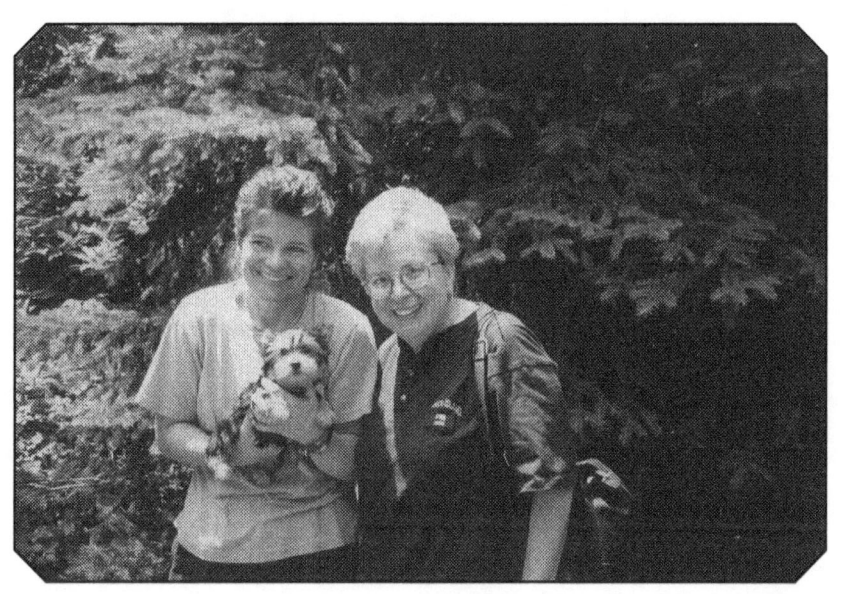

CHERYL WITH LYSE AND MOLLY

The wind knows no pain
Running through heartaches
Singing of memories

Cheryl L. Cushine

www.ingramcontent.com/pod-product-compliance
Lightning Source LLC
Chambersburg PA
CBHW061312280526
45784CB00002B/962